SIMON & SCHUSTER

Dear Reader,

Su Meck is quite possibly the most remarkable woman I've ever met.

Though she's in her forties now, the day Su came to New York to meet with publishers was the first time she'd ever traveled alone. More than twenty-five years after the accident that left her with a traumatic brain injury (TBI) and complete retrograde amnesia, she had still felt the need to tape a note to the mirror in her hotel room reminding her who and where she was in case she woke up disoriented.

The more I learned of Su's story, the more I was stunned by the scope of the challenges she had faced: How do you raise children when you have no memory of being parented yourself? How do you maintain a relationship with your husband when you've forgotten everything you once knew about love and sex? And yet despite this kind of daily struggle, Su has raised three charming and successful children. She has become an accomplished drummer and author, and just a few months after this book is published, she will receive a bachelor's degree from one of the most prestigious women's colleges in the country.

I Forgot to Remember is a memoir about loss and restoration, a raw and fearless account of what can happen when the things we once thought defined us—our histories, our personalities, our culture—are taken away. In her own indelible voice, Su offers us a view from the inside of a terrible injury, with the hope that her story will help give other TBI sufferers and their families the resolve and courage to build their lives anew. Piercing, heartbreaking, but finally uplifting, this book is the true story of a woman determined to live life on her own terms.

I hope you'll be as inspired by Su's story as I am, and would love to hear your thoughts.

All best,

Molly Lindley | Associate Editor | (212) 698-7342 | molly.lindley@simonandschuster.com

A Memoir of Amnesia

~

I Forgot to Remember

Su Meck

with Daniel de Visé

Simon & Schuster

New York London Toronto Sydney New Delhi

Simon & Schuster
1230 Avenue of the Americas
New York, NY 10020

First Simon & Schuster hardcover edition February 2014

For information about special discounts for bulk purchases, please contact Simon & Schuster Special Sales at 1-866-506-1949 or business@simonandschuster.com.

The Simon & Schuster Speakers Bureau can bring authors to your live event. For more information or to book an event contact the Simon & Schuster Speakers Bureau at 1-866-248-3049 or visit our website at www.simonspeakers.com.

Manufactured in the United States of America

1 3 5 7 9 10 8 6 4 2

Library of Congress Cataloging-in-Publication Data Tk

ISBN 978-1-4516-8581-7
ISBN 978-1-4516-8583-1 (ebook)

To Mom and Dad for giving me life

To Benjamin, Patrick, and Kassidy for patiently teaching me about life and guiding me so lovingly through life

To Jim for enabling me, even encouraging me,
to share with the world so much about this, our crazy life

I sincerely hope some good can come from all of this,
especially for those with TBI, their families, and their friends.

These Are the Days of Our Lives

—Queen

I never had aspirations as a writer. But here I am, writing. I was a difficult child. But evidently I wasn't all that different from most other children growing up in the 1960s and 70s. I lacked motivation in school. And yet report cards show me to be an excellent student. I got drunk a lot as a teenager but I have never tasted alcohol. I have no idea what falling in love feels like, and yet I have been married for almost thirty years.

These examples are just a small sampling of the many inconsistencies that make up my life as I know it. Actually, my lives. I have at least two of them. My first life began when I was born in the summer of 1965 and progressed through until the spring of 1988. I do not have any genuine memories from any of this first life. Then there is the life I mostly remember living since roughly 1991 or 1992. But I have discovered recently that I have several other "lives" as well. Because I depend solely on the stories of others to fill in decades of living, anecdotes about who I was, what I did, and how I lived, I have found that my life story varies depending on whom I talk to. And a lot of the time, accounts of a certain event don't just differ, instead they totally contradict each other.

I had no idea how much this life of mine would transform when I first began telling my story. After Daniel de Visé's article about me appeared in the Sunday edition *Washington Post,* on May 21, 2011 suddenly my family and I were big news. I became kind of a poster child for traumatic brain injury (TBI). People wanted to interview me on both the radio and television. I received hundreds of e-mails from people living all over the world relating their own struggles living with TBI, and telling me that my story gave them hope.

Literary agents began contacting me asking if I would be willing to write a memoir, and at first the thought of writing a book seemed preposterous to me. But as I read about the hopes, as well as the frustrations, of other people who were reaching out to me, it suddenly dawned on me that maybe telling my story could help get the word out about what it is like to live in an often confusing world, made even more confusing because of a baffling brain injury.

However, if I agreed to write my story, I wanted to make sure that I would be able to tell the whole sordid tale, not only with my family's permission but with their blessing as well. This story is not some kind of fairy tale that begins with "once upon a time" and ends with "and everyone lived happily ever after." I wanted to write truth. And that's when it began to get tricky. As my husband,

Jim, and I like to say, the whole thing was a mission "fraught with peril." How is someone like me, with no memories of at least the first twentysomething years of her life, supposed to write a memoir? And how are friends and family in the year 2013 supposed to remember exactly what I was like and what I was doing in 1965? 1972? 1980? How are those same friends and family members supposed to remember what exactly happened on a Sunday afternoon in May of 1988?

With the help of Daniel de Visé, I was able to track down my medical records from the hospital in Fort Worth, Texas. Dan agreed to undertake the job of researcher, investigating some of the medical breakthroughs that have been made in the science of the brain since the 1980s, as well as brain conditions that continue to baffle the medical community. He then sifted through all of those details, and made an attempt to explain them to me. In addition, I have spoken with many people who knew me as I was growing up. I have had long conversations with my parents and siblings, as well as other close family members and friends.

It is difficult for me to be so unbelievably dependent on stories about myself from other people as I try to get to the truth about my life. Part of me realizes that I will never really know exactly what I was like before my head injury, or understand why I am the way I am now. But another part of me stubbornly refuses to give up as I try desperately to fit pieces together in an ever-changing life-size puzzle.

1

Life in the Fast Lane

—Eagles

I don't remember any of what I'm about to tell you. Sure, I know the story, but it *is* just a story related to me by others, in bits and pieces, over many years. I have attempted to collect those scraps in order to present a narrative that feels real and whole. But it has been difficult. I have had to interpret the story, to picture the scenes in my mind, just as you are about to do. Some of the pieces are missing, because the people who witnessed them have forgotten the details, or because the people have themselves disappeared. Part of what continues to be maddening for me is the number of questions I still have that nobody seems to be able to answer in any kind of satisfactory way. Imagine the defining day of your life, stitched together from other people's memories.

This story starts on May 22, 1988. It is important to appreciate that what happened on that day was quite literally life changing for many people. Not just me. As I write about what transpired, I will rely chiefly on the memories of my husband, Jim, the only living soul who was present on that day and can recount what happened. Or at least how he remembers it happening. I was there, too, of course, but my memories are lost. My two sons were there, but they were too young to remember what took place that day.

This was the day that my old life ended and my new life began. I died, in a way, and was reborn, with the same physical form, but not the same mind. My body still knew how to do a few of the things I had taught it to do, like play the drums and ride a bicycle. But that's where the similarities end. The two Sus have lived separate lives. She never knew me, and I know nothing of her except what people have told me. She rebelled; I conform. She broke rules; I follow them. She drank and smoked pot; I don't even know the taste of beer or wine, and the smell of smoke makes me physically ill. I like vegetables; she hated them. She loved to swim; I am absolutely terrified of the water.

I still to this day sit around with my family and listen to stories about the other Su, in the same way that a child might sit and hear of things that happened before she was born. Our family history has two distinct chapters, *Before Su* and *After Su*. My husband, being a computer geek, sometimes calls me Su 2.0.

You might wonder how it feels to wake up one morning and not know who you are. I don't know. The accident didn't just wipe out all my memories; it hindered me from making new ones for quite some time. I awoke each day to a house full of strangers. Every morning began with a lesson: *Welcome to your new life.* And this wasn't just a few days. It was weeks before I recognized my boys

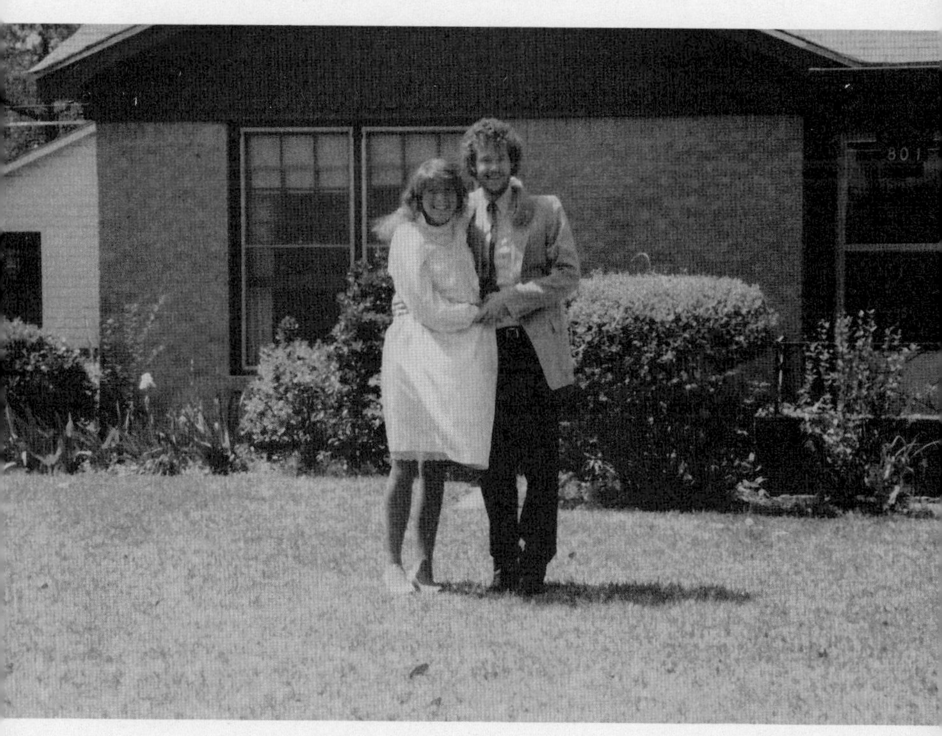

Jim and me in Texas, spring 1986. I am pregnant with Benjamin.

when they toddled into the room, months before I knew my own telephone number, years before I was able to find my way home from anywhere. I have no more memory of those first several years after the accident than my own kids have of their first years of life.

For years, I didn't even know the exact date that the accident happened. Isn't that sad, not knowing the precise moment when your life changed forever? All I knew, or thought I knew, was that it was a February afternoon in 1988. Jim thought it was a weekday. All of those details and facts turned out to be wrong. The hospital records, when we finally got them, put the date at May 22, a Sunday, three days before Jim's and my third wedding anniversary.

That particular day started out as a very typical Sunday in the Meck home. The first nine hours of that day were so routine, in fact, that there's not much Jim remembers for certain. When people remember stuff, it's usually the remarkable or shocking things, and the first part of that day was utterly unremarkable. It's the events from later in the day that are unforgettable. Well, not for me. And try to keep in mind that every memory from Jim is scarred by panic, pain, and loss.

Here, then, is what would have happened on a typical Sunday for me in the spring of 1988. I can't stress enough that this is not a factual account of what transpired the day, but merely an educated guess.

I awoke that morning tangled up in candy-striped flannel sheets on our king-size waterbed. Warm Texas sunshine was already streaming through the arched Spanish-style window of the bedroom, making a crisscross shadow pattern of the decorative wrought-iron bars on our beige carpet.

As I lay in that place halfway between sleep and wakefulness, I looked around the white-walled room and took stock of the facts:

I was only twenty-two, and already twice a college dropout, thrust into the routines of marriage and motherhood, transplanted from Main Line Philadelphia to a faceless working-class suburb of Fort Worth. Next to me lay Jim, my husband and the father of my two baby boys. Benjamin, just shy of his second birthday, was sleeping in a twin bed in his room, beneath a dinosaur comforter. Patrick, at eight months, slept in his crib in the tiny third bedroom. Because it was a Sunday, Jim and I would head to church with the boys in a few hours. But first, if our early-morning whispers with each other did not wake the boys, Jim and I may have quickly and quietly made love. Afterward, we may have talked about plans for our wedding anniversary as well as Benjamin's second birthday. Both were coming up. Our anniversary was in just three days. Were reservations already made for fancy dinner out? Did we have a babysitter lined up? Did we exchange cards? Gifts? Benjamin's birthday was only ten days away. Were there birthday gifts for him already bought, wrapped, and hidden away somewhere? Had I sent birthday party invitations to a bunch of the neighborhood kids? Or maybe that's exactly what I was going to do after church that day.

We eventually got up and padded off to the shower together, tiptoeing across the worn carpet on soft feet, still trying our best not to wake the boys. After showers and dressing, I poked my head into Benjamin's room to get him up and going before heading to change Patrick's diaper and get him his morning bottle. As I carried Patrick toward the kitchen, I couldn't help but glance at the walls in the hallway lined with dozens of framed photos of our young family: Benjamin being held by my parents, dressed in his white baptismal outfit; another of Benjamin, sleeping facedown in his cake on his first birthday; Jim and me out in Middle-of-Nowhere, Texas, holding hands with strangers during Hands

Jim and I sang the hymns, recited readings, prayed, and listened to the sermon, something I can't even imagine now. Church is one of those things that the new me has never quite figured out. I still don't fully understand the endless monologues about this man named Jesus who lives everywhere while being invisible, who is dead but still alive, both father and son. I have no idea if I in fact had faith or even believed in God before. But after the accident, I found myself wishing that instead of having to sit through an hour-long church service, I could instead slip away and join my sons in their Sunday school classrooms, where perhaps things were explained a bit more clearly.

After church, we returned home to our ranch house on El Greco Avenue, a tiny house with the water heater tucked right inside the front hall closet to save space. I cannot recall that house on El Greco, but Jim has shown me pictures. It was a tract home in a working-class neighborhood called Wedgwood, south of downtown Fort Worth. All the homes in that neighborhood, constructed in the early 1970s, were built for first-time homeowners. It was a neighborhood of pregnant moms and strollers, older station wagons, and backyard barbecues. Our house at 6609 El Greco was indistinguishable from all the others. There was a house just like ours to the left, and another on our right. We moved into it in 1987, hoping to settle down and stay put after five moves in and around Fort Worth just two years.

It was my habit in those days to sit outside on the ribbed, folding lawn chair on our back patio with a fresh legal pad for a Sunday-afternoon routine of letter writing while the kids played in the yard. I was a good writer back then, with a broad vocabulary of SAT words and a confident, flowing script. Family and friends all lived far away from us, so I regularly included updated photos of the boys in my letters. One letter for my parents, one for my grandparents, letters for my brothers and sisters, possibly one for my high school friend Kathy and another for Michele, my college roommate. One for each of the people I was about to forget.

~

When I was in high school I lived with my family in a wealthy Philadelphia suburb. I wanted for nothing. My father was a chemical engineer, my mother an overachieving stay-at-home mom who did more in five minutes than most moms accomplished in a whole day. I was made in their image, with a clever mind, musical talent, an athletic body, and a determined, but reasonably stubborn personality.

But I ended up labeled as the Millers' rebellious child. In fifth grade, when I was asked to pick a musical instrument, I chose the drums. In high school, I drank, smoked pot, and partied, though I still managed to earn mostly A's and B's. I went to college at Ohio Wesleyan University, a private liberal arts school, with a pretty campus in the town of Delaware, just north of Columbus. At the beginning of my sophomore year, I got pregnant and had an abortion. At the end of my sophomore year, I dropped out of college, got married, moved to Texas, started school at Texas Christian University, got pregnant again, and dropped out again, all by the age of twenty.

I married at nineteen, younger than my daughter, Kassidy, is now. My parents apparently couldn't stop me. I sure as hell would stop her. Or at least I hope I would. What was it about me that couldn't be stopped? What about me was so uncontrollable? To run off and get married at nineteen? I would go to the ends of the earth before I would let my daughter do that. What about me

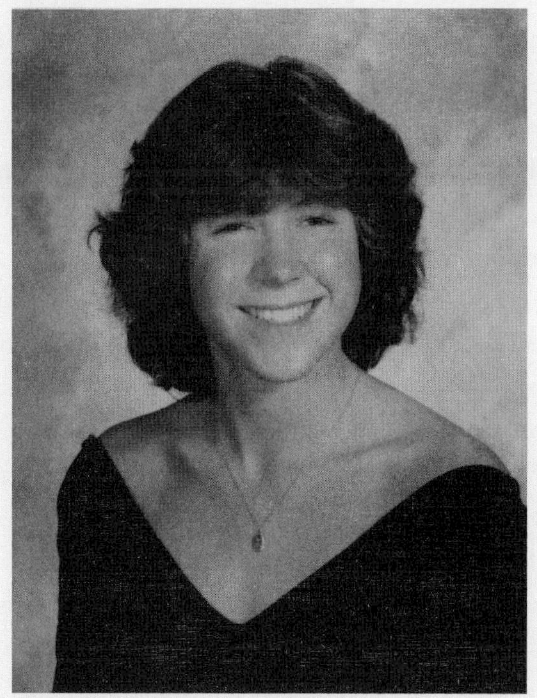

My Conestoga High School senior portrait that was used in the freshman *Look Book* at Ohio Wesleyan University in fall 1983.

could my parents not stop? That's a big question for me now, and I don't have an answer. Nobody does.

I met Jim at Ohio Wesleyan my freshman year. He was a junior and had seen me in the *OWU Look Book,* the book put out by the school with all the pictures of new freshman and transfer students, in the fall of 1983. He walked up to me at a band practice that September and said, "Oh, hi, you must be Su. You're a freshman here, right?" He says I looked at him as if he was dog shit I just had scraped off my shoe. Both of us were in other relationships. But late that fall we ended up in a car together on a weekend canoe outing with his fraternity and my sorority. On the way back, in a Wendy's drive-through, he kissed me.

Four years later, Jim was a twenty-four-year-old software engineer at General Dynamics, a campus of forty thousand workers across from Carswell Air Force Base, and part of the Strategic Air Command. GD and Carswell AFB were cogs in the tank-tread wheels of the old Cold War America. He left at 7:15 each morning in jeans, loafers, and a polo shirt and spent his days writing software for F-16 fighter jets. Many of our neighbors were young single-income families whose husbands and fathers also worked at General Dynamics. Mike and Pam Knote, for example, lived right across the street, and were only a few years older than we were, with two boys of their own, a five-year-old and a toddler. Mike Knote went off to work at General Dynamics every day, just like Jim. Pam stayed home, just like me.

During the day, Jim and I seldom spoke to each other. His scheduled work hours usually ended at four, but most days he worked late into the evenings in order to get the overtime. So I never really knew when he was going to arrive home. He didn't like me to call him at work, but I was okay with that. I was happy to sit

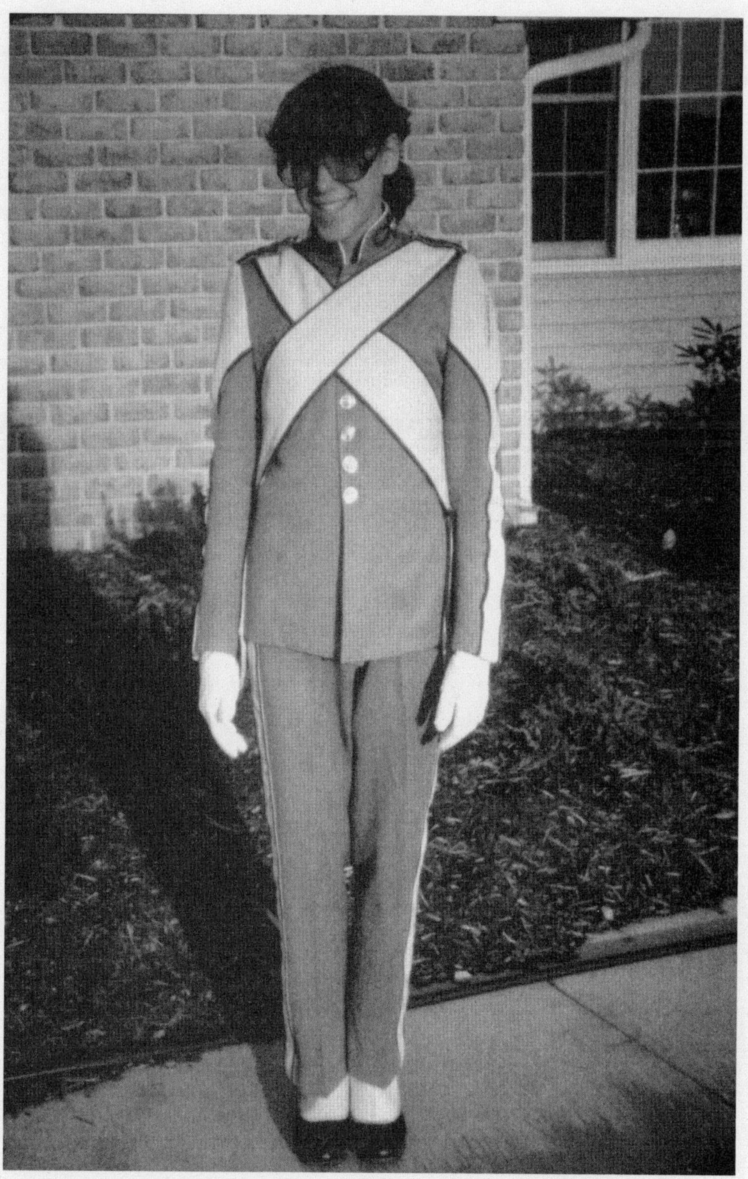

I was a drummer in the Conestoga High School Pioneer Marching Band during the golden years of the early 1980s.

at home and wait to eat with him after feeding the boys their supper. The evening entertainment was usually books or a video. And there was always music playing.

I loved rock-and-roll music, mostly from the 1960s and 70s, as well as all the great current 1980s stuff. I still have all of my old vinyl records and a huge cassette-tape collection. More than anything, I liked and often played along with my favorite drummers: Neil Peart, from Rush, Keith Moon from the Who, Nick Mason from Pink Floyd, John Bonham from Led Zep, and, of course, Ringo. Unfortunately, we ended up having to sell my drum kit early in our marriage. There were bills to pay. After the accident, Jim remembers me putting on records and dancing around the living room with the boys. Maybe we did that before the accident, too. Maybe we had danced around the living room on that very Sunday afternoon in May.

We had resided in the house on El Greco for less than a year, but Jim already knew the way to the hospital. I was apparently accident-prone. Less than three years earlier, at our wedding, my father had taken Jim aside and told him, "Find the nearest emergency room as soon as you get to Texas, because about every six months, Su finds a need to be there."

In our short time living on El Greco, I had already proven him right. Eight months earlier, a fierce bout of influenza had sent me into early labor. Patrick was born in the hospital downtown, a month premature and weighing not quite four pounds. We called him our little spider monkey. A few months after that, Benjamin, while throwing a typical eighteen-month-old temper tantrum, had hurled a heavy wooden Playskool truck through the window in our bedroom, creating a hole the size of a volleyball in the glass. Impulsive and impatient, I reached through the broken glass to pick up the truck and somehow managed to slice through the webbing between my thumb and forefinger, badly injuring my hand. When I couldn't get the bleeding to stop on my own, I called Jim. He drove right home and took me to the ER. I ended up needing nineteen stitches both inside my hand and out.

~

As we settled into our evening routine on that Sunday in May, Jim thinks that he and I talked about the possibility of renting a movie after the kids had gone to bed. Then our thoughts turned to, "What shall we eat for dinner?"

Later I was clattering around the electric stove making macaroni and cheese, adding dollops of Velveeta to the pot because that was the way Benjamin liked it, smooth and creamy with no lumps. I may have been planning to boil some peas in another pot. Jim sat at the kitchen table, reading the Sunday edition of the *Fort Worth Star Telegram* and playing the part of suburban dad. Benjamin sat in his high chair eating Cheerios. I may have also been fixing a bottle of milk for Patrick, who was crawling around entertaining himself with his toys on the carpet in the family room right off the kitchen.

It's the next moment when Jim's memories come into sharp focus. He distinctly remembers seeing Patrick out of the corner of his eye, crawling between the dark wooden spindles of the railing that separated the family room from the kitchen.

Nobody knows what exactly happened next. Jim's back was turned. "I hear this noise," Jim recalls. "I have only an auditory memory of what it sounded like. I remember being startled. I turn, and this is the picture: it's something out of the movie *Carrie*, where I'm standing, I'm turning, you're holding out Patrick, and as you're handing him to me, you're collapsing, blood flowing from your head down your front." As I crumpled to the floor, Jim says he watched the light in my eyes go out.

For a few seconds, Jim just stood there, his mind not yet comprehending what had happened.

"I'm trying to figure out what to do next," he recalls, "because what I'm seeing makes no sense."

My body lay on the floor in a heap, inert. The ceiling fan hovered a foot or so above me. Somehow, those facts were connected.

Jim's moment of paralysis passed. He stepped around my fallen body and the swaying ceiling fan and crossed the kitchen to the telephone hanging on the wall just around the corner. With Patrick in one arm and the phone in the other, he dialed 911.

"Nine-one-one. What is your emergency?"

"I'm in my house. My wife has collapsed."

"All right, sir. Is she breathing?"

"I don't know."

"All right, sir. We'll get someone there as soon as we can."

Patrick's voice had risen to a wail, and by the end of the call, Jim was shouting over it. Jim gave the dispatcher our address and hung up the phone. Benjamin sat in his high chair, speechless, his eyes fixed on the floor where his mommy lay.

Jim stood in the kitchen and studied the scene. I lay on the floor, a pool of blood expanding outward from the gash in my forehead. Above my limp body swung the ceiling fan, now freakishly suspended by a frayed cord. Jim's eyes followed the cord to the ceiling and saw the bare hook that had once held it sticking out from a ragged hole in the plaster. I wonder now about that fan. Were there any other exposed wires hanging down? Was it a fire hazard? Wasn't Jim worried about himself or the boys getting electrocuted? How could he have left it hanging there? How is it that the oddly dangling fan could have been ignored?

The fan had come with the house. Nothing in its previous behavior had given us cause for alarm. It was quiet, well balanced, and it had always cooled the kitchen nicely.

For a few moments, panic receded and Jim's engineer brain asserted itself. He pieced together what he thinks might have happened: "I thought back, and I can remember you saying, 'Weeee,'" Jim recalls, reenacting the scene for me with a pillow. "And I'm thinking, so, you walked over to Patrick and said, 'Weeee,' and picked him up. As you held him up, over your head, either his back, or his feet hit the fan, and it came crashing down on you."

I have often thought about Patrick: By what miracle was he totally unharmed? How is it the fan did not hit him? How was it that I was able to hand him to Jim before collapsing? And what about Benjamin? Jim says he was right there, sitting in his high chair. What did he see? His mom lying on the floor, in a pool of blood? How awful would that be for him? Thankfully, he says he doesn't remember anything about that day.

Jim considered what to do next. He knew enough first aid to know not to try to move me. He thought, Okay, the ambulance is coming and they're going to take you. I need to figure out somewhere for the boys to be. He scooped them up and dashed across the street to the Knotes, our neighbors and friends.

Pam Knote opened the door. Jim said, "There's been an accident. The ambulance is coming. Can I leave the guys with you?"

Pam recalls that Jim looked "calm but frantic, you know, very urgent." The tone in his voice told her there was no time to explain.

"I mostly remember him just handing me Patrick." She left all four kids with her husband, Mike, and set off across the street with Jim to put together a diaper bag.

An ambulance had arrived by this point and now sat parked outside our home; Jim and Pam walked in to find two paramedics tending to me. "You were lying on the kitchen floor," Pam recalls. "There was blood on your face and under your head. The paramedics were asking you some questions, and you were able to respond, but I don't know how coherent you were."

Pam too remembers seeing the ceiling fan dangling near the floor. She also saw, protruding from the ceiling, "a hook with a lip on it that should have been up in the ceiling but wasn't." As she took in the scene, she marveled that I had somehow managed to keep the fan from hurting my baby. "That was your first instinct as a mom," Pam remembers thinking to herself, "to protect Patrick." Pam collected diapers, bottles, blankets, and changes of clothing, stuffed everything into a bag, and headed back across the street to Benjamin and Patrick, leaving Jim to stay with me.

Jim hovered over the paramedics. One looked up, gestured across the room, and said, "Sir, please stand over there and stay out of our way."

A paramedic shined a bright pen light into my pupils. One of them had shrunk to a pinprick; the other had swelled. Neither one responded to the light the way it should. Jim watched the men stick pins in my fingers and then heard one of them say, "She's completely unresponsive."

Was I awake? Jim and Pam's accounts differ on this point. Pam says she remembers me speaking to the paramedics. But is she really just remembering them speaking to me? Jim says he doesn't remember hearing my voice or seeing me stir at any point, not in the seven minutes from when the fan hit me till the paramedics arrived, nor in the ten minutes from their arrival until my body was whisked away on a backboard. But his memories of that day are colored by panic and shock. When he heard the paramedics say, "She's completely unresponsive," did they mean that I was out cold, or merely that some of my fingers and toes were numb and failing to react to the prick of a pin?

A second rescue unit pulled up; this one was a full-size fire truck. An incident commander entered the house with two or three other men in heavy fire jackets and hats. Two of them carried a backboard that was meant for me.

A big red fire engine with flashing lights and firefighters rushing around in jackets and hats must have made for quite a scene outside the door of our little home. Did our neighbors step outside to see what was going on? Did they stay indoors and peer through curtains? Did other people on El Greco wonder what could have drawn the Fort Worth Fire Department to the Mecks' door? Did they care?

Inside our house no one was talking much, but Jim remembers glimpsing the frequent nonverbal cues passed back and forth between the commander and the paramedics, a faint shaking of heads and furrowing of brows, all seeding a sense of foreboding. "I remember them being very grim," Jim recalls. "You know: it just did not look good, not good at all."

The paramedics bandaged an inch-long gash on my forehead: such a small wound, but so much blood, pooling in a three-foot diameter around my head. Workers carefully fitted a cervical brace around my neck. Then several of them encircled me and ever so gently lifted me onto the backboard. They strapped my body to the board and rushed out of the house to load me into the ambulance.

Jim asked if he could come along. "No, sir," a paramedic told him, "you can't go in the ambulance. We aren't covered for that."

The ambulance door swung closed, and I began my journey to the hospital. I would like to tell you that the paramedic gazed pensively at my vital signs, steadied my wounded head, held my hand, and even though I couldn't hear the words, he told me in a thick Texas accent, "Everything's gonna be just fine." But Jim wasn't there, and I don't remember, so there is nothing more to tell.

2

Confusion

—ELO

I have read through all of the medical records of my stay in the hospital and, quite honestly, I haven't a clue as to what much of it means. There seems to be a lot of secret medical language that us patient types aren't meant to understand. But I do, unfortunately, notice plenty of discrepancies among the hundreds of pages of records from the hospital. In the notes from one doctor on May 25, 1988, it says that the ceiling fan struck me on the left temple, but I was actually hit on the right side. There are accounts written about my condition on June 9 describing my impaired memory, impaired communication, dysfunctional mobility, impaired judgment, and decreased attention span, and yet I was discharged the very next day. It was noted on May 31 that my long-term memory "seems fairly unaffected." (Really? Hmm. Interesting.) There are several pages included in my records that aren't even mine.

I guess I expected, and was hoping, for those records to somehow hold *the key* that would give me answers and fill in gaps. I was hoping that these *official records* would be just that. Instead, the written record just raises even more questions about why I am the way I am, and what the medical community did and did not do when I was first injured. It is difficult for me to piece together all of the facts of my stay in the hospital from these discombobulated accounts, but I will do my best.

~

Jim always talks about how after I was whisked away in the ambulance, he can remember climbing into his powder-blue Chevy Malibu in our driveway. But he doesn't remember the drive to the hospital. He always says that he arrived before the ambulance, ruining his car's transmission in the process.

My records show that I was registered into Harris Methodist Southwest Hospital at 6:30 P.M., a Caucasian female, age twenty-two, of Presbyterian faith. The diagnosis, in capital letters: "CEILING FAN FELL ON HEAD." The bottom of the page bears my husband's hurried signature: James R. Meck.

Jim thinks he phoned his parents, and then my parents, calling collect. Remember this was the 1980s, and there were no cell phones. My mom recalls the conversation this way: "Jim said that you had had an accident. And I said, 'What now?' I had to ask him that because you were always such a rambunctious daredevil." (I have since heard stories of my childhood escapades—tumbling off trampolines, plummeting headlong out of trees, and careening down steep hills in wagons.) Mom continues: "And I just remember Jim saying, 'I need your help, it's really serious this time.' "

There is a moment from that evening that Jim recalls sitting alone in the waiting room. Waiting. He watched the sunset out the window, and gazed across the newly developed area of suburban Fort Worth. "My mind was racing, trying to think of anything and everything that could be done," he remembers. "This was before the Internet. All I had was what was between my ears." And as he sat there thinking, it struck him how alone he and I were. My parents and younger brother were in Houston, four or five hours away. His family was in Georgia. "There was this profound sense of dread and loneliness, or aloneness," he recalls. "There wasn't anything to do, and yet there was a huge motivation to *do* something."

Because there was nothing else to do, and Jim was tired of sitting, he pestered the duty nurse every few minutes. Finally, a physician emerged. He told Jim that I was stable but comatose, and partly paralyzed on my left side. Fluid was pressing against the inside of my skull, but if doctors attempted surgery to relieve the pressure, there was a good chance the pressure would cause my brain to burst. Not a happy thought. The doctor explained that the brain floats in fluid, and a sac holds it in place, sort of like a parachute. The impact of the fan, he said, had set off a chain of events: the front of my brain had struck the front of my skull, and then it had bounced back, and the back of my brain had struck the back of my skull. The doctor continued, "Imagine if you ever put Jell-O in a fridge, and you take it out and you shake it, and there's cracks in it. That's what happened to your wife's brain."

Then he told Jim that there was nothing more he could do, which Jim didn't appreciate. "I'm a systems engineer. We systems guys fix stuff. There are always things you do, and if one thing doesn't work, you do the next thing." It was just inconceivable to Jim, and frankly, he found it irresponsible, that they would do nothing. It seemed like a cop-out. It was as though they were only worried about covering their asses rather than doing something in order to help me. Jim got hot. He lost his temper and became verbally abusive. He says he can remember distinctly challenging the doctor and nurses, screaming at everyone: "What do you mean you can't do anything? What is your medical degree worth? Because right now you're doing nothing." He doesn't remember what else he said. "To their credit, they didn't have me arrested. And in retrospect, it's the only reason you are still alive, because they did nothing."

A decision was made to move me from Harris Methodist Southwest to Harris Methodist, a sister facility in downtown Fort Worth with a comprehensive neurological intensive care unit. I often wonder if Jim's ranting and raving had anything to do with why I was moved. But Jim recalls "having a feeling in the back of my head that they were overwhelmed" [at Harris Methodist Southwest], and they couldn't handle my situation. Regardless, the people working in that emergency room were probably glad to see me transferred. And Jim along with me.

~

The discharge papers from the first hospital listed my condition as poor, and to Jim's eye I looked like I was getting worse. I was more pale and fragile-looking. The transfer was a delicate maneuver. At the downtown hospital, another very calm, very senior nurse asked Jim to recount what had happened. When the narrative got to Patrick, and to the fact that it was his little body that had struck the fan, the nurse suddenly grew alarmed. Patrick had, after all, been in the same accident as I had. "Where is Patrick now?" she asked. "Who checked him out?" No one had. She said, "We'll get the rest of this information later. Go now and get your son." Jim drove home to get Patrick from the Knotes' house. When he arrived back at the hospital, Patrick was rushed to the pediatric ER for a battery of tests. He had a small scrape on his cheek, but thankfully nothing worse.

Jim was told that one of the hospital's top neurosurgeons was coming on duty at midnight. This doctor was said to be brilliant, but antisocial, even kind of reclusive. "He asks for the night shift," one doctor told Jim, "because he doesn't like talking to people. Don't expect a lot of bedside manner. But trust me, he's as good as we have for making this kind of neurological call."

At 11 P.M., a nurse at Harris Methodist examined me. Her notes state that I did not lose consciousness immediately upon being hit on the head, but passed out shortly thereafter. A subsequent note states that I lost consciousness "approximately three minutes post-injury" and remained out "for about five minutes." Another note from that night states, "Patient is easily aroused but drowsy," and is "oriented to space and time." Yet another note says: "Patient's left arm feels "funny," her left leg feels "heavy," and her head hurts "inside."

At 11:20 P.M., the famed antisocial neurosurgeon arrived. Dr. Joe Ellis Wheeler was middle-aged, balding and portly, with pasty skin, salt-and-pepper hair, and piercing blue eyes. He examined me. Then he called Jim into his office.

"There was a pipe smell," Jim recalls. "A wall of leather-bound books. A great intelligence was there. He sounded like someone who had an absolute command of his field. Here was somebody I implicitly trusted."

Dr. Wheeler told Jim that I had suffered a closed-head injury, affecting not my skull but the soft tissue inside. X-rays showed no fractured skull, no compressed vertebrae. Jim asked him what could be done. Dr. Wheeler said, "The fluid is what's killing your wife. If we opened her skull, because of the pressure inside, the result would just be catastrophic. The best thing we can do is just withdraw all treatments, the fluids, the IV, so the tissues can naturally reabsorb the fluids in her head. We need to give her body a chance to absorb the trauma." Jim remembers Dr. Wheeler saying this, too: "I'll be honest with you: most people with this level of internal injury do not survive."

Jim made another round of collect calls to his family and mine. He told them, "They've convinced me that the best course of action is to do nothing. We'll have to wait it out." He recalls saying, too, that I "had a chance of recovering, but it's only a chance. I wasn't trying to sugarcoat anything. I thought you were dying. There was desperation on the other end of the phone, once we got past 'Can we come? Can we be there?' Because there was no physical way to get from A to B. Everybody was going to check what flights there were in the morning, but there was nothing that could be done right then," Jim says. "And you might not be there in the morning."

My mom doesn't recall any such dire language from Jim: "He didn't say, 'This is so serious the whole family should gather around right now.' " Although Mom being Mom, she may have just heard those words and gone into a kind of motherly denial. I know that may sound harsh, but my mom tends to occasionally understand things to be the way she wants them to be rather than the way they actually are. In any event, no one was close enough to climb into a car and drive to the hospital at that late hour.

Nurses kept bringing Jim things: coffee, and little cups of ice cream. They kept coaxing him to leave: "Mr. Meck, we'll let you know." Jim stayed. "I was concerned that you would die, and I wouldn't be there."

A nurse filled out a personal data form on me at 1:15 A.M., probably with Jim's help. The form lists each of my previous hospitalizations. Though I was only twenty-two, there weren't enough lines on the form to list them all: major knee surgery, 1981; elective abortion, 1984; ovarian cysts, 1984; miscarriage, 1985; childbirth by cesarean section, 1986 and 1987; hand injury, 1987. Jim signed some more papers, permitting the doctors to remove the intravenous tubes from my veins. He says Dr. Wheeler told him, "You should get your sons and say good-bye." So he did.

By this time it was very late. During the drive back to the hospital, both Benjamin and Patrick fell fast asleep. Jim parked the car, and carried the boys to my hospital room in the ICU. It was quiet. The doctors had turned everything off. I lay on the hospital bed, pale and still, my head bandaged. The rhythmic beat of a heart monitor and my breathing were the only sounds in the room. "You were sweaty, hair stringing down over your face, bandages on your head, blotchy, kind of waxy," Jim recalls. "It was like you weren't you. It was like you had already gone." And in a way I had.

Jim pondered what to do, and he made a decision. "It was so late and I couldn't wake up Benjamin or Patrick," he recalled. "And I couldn't say good-bye. I was all ready to because of what the doctor had told me. But I had these angelic guys in my arms, and I decided, 'I'm not going to wake you, and I'm not going to say good-bye.' " Jim hugged his sons, and then leaned each sleepy baby over to press their lips against my cheek. "And then I kissed you, and we left."

On the drive home, Jim recalls, "The anger and the frustration had burned themselves out. So I guess at this point I was just tired and resigned and there was just a tremendous feeling of loss. He doesn't recall thinking, " 'How did this happen to me, how did this happen to us?' Instead there was just grief and loss." Jim vividly does remember making a plea, repeating it over and over in his head: "If there's any way that Su can get through this, I'll do anything." It wasn't a prayer to God exactly, Jim says, instead it was just "a promise I was making," maybe just a promise to himself. Little did he realize precisely what he was asking. There is a saying: Be careful what you wish for, because you might get it.

Jim remembers parking his sick car in the driveway and walking into the house. The kitchen was just as the paramedics had left it, the fan still dangling from the ceiling, the blood still pooled on the floor. He put the boys to bed, and then he picked up the bandages and wrappings and discarded IVs. He searched around and finally found a bucket and a sponge and set about cleaning the pooled blood from the kitchen floor. He remembers that, with every sweep of the sponge, the circle of blood seemed to grow larger. "It was like a metaphor for the idea that nothing I did seemed to make a difference," he recalls. After cleaning up the kitchen as best as he could, he removed his red-stained jeans and polo shirt and took a long, hot shower, washing his wife's blood from his hands and arms and knees. Then he fell into bed.

~

Back at the hospital, in the intensive care unit, nurses made hourly entries on my progress:

> 1:15: Alert but lethargic, and poorly responding to orientation questions.
>
> 2:00: Severe headache. Wiggles both legs on command.
>
> 3:30: Darvocet for headache.
>
> 4:30: Patient has started menstruating. Pupils unequal. Verbalizing more freely and asking appropriate questions.
>
> 5:30: More photophobic than earlier. Hand grip still very weak.

~

A cinematic version of my story might have me open my eyes, wince at the pain of the morning sun, and survey my surroundings in blank wonder. In fact, I appear to have spent my first twenty-four hours in the hospital much like most ICU patients do, in a blur of wakefulness and sleep. In those first waking moments, as I surveyed myself and my surroundings, no one—least of all me—knows what thoughts entered my mind, if any. Most likely, I didn't know who I was, or where I was, or why I was there. I probably didn't recognize my own arms and legs, or the television hanging from the wall, or the window, or the door. Everything would have been unfamiliar.

So many questions occurred to me as I read through all of these entries in my medical records. How can someone be *alert* and *lethargic* at the same time? Did I know what *menstruating* was? Did I even notice? How exactly was I verbalizing? What *appropriate* questions did I ask? Did I know enough to grasp that I was even supposed to know who I was, and where I was, and what the names of the items in my room were, and what purpose they served? I was, in all probability, as bewildered as a newborn.

That morning was Monday, May 23. When Jim arrived at the hospital, he spoke to the duty nurse and learned that I had survived the night. "The worst had passed, for me, at that moment," he recalls. "My prayers had been answered. However, I had no idea what was coming."

But another nurse gently prepared him: "Your wife doesn't know her name." Jim walked into my room where the lights had been dimmed to ease the pain in my head. He greeted me. He says he knew right away that I didn't recognize him. I looked at him, but I did not reward him, or anyone else, with so much as a flash of recognition. But at that moment Jim was preoccupied by the simple fact that I was alive.

"I guess I was so relieved that you were breathing and opening your eyes that it didn't hit me until later that something was profoundly wrong," he recalls. "It hadn't sunk in yet, the extent to which you weren't really there. I didn't even think about it. You woke up. So to me it wasn't like there had been any loss."

Dr. Wheeler, the ace neurosurgeon, had left a report. It said I had stabilized; there was no need for surgery. Jim called his parents again, and mine: "The worst has passed. She's still here." I am still not at all convinced that anybody had a clue how bad the worst had been. Or would be.

~

The formal diagnosis from Dr. Wheeler states that I suffered a "minor closed-head injury" and a "possible cerebral concussion," neither of which sounded very bad. Dr. Wheeler gives a similarly muted account of the injury: "When the patient was first struck on the head, [she] was not immediately knocked out, but became drowsy, nauseated, and she complained of a funny feeling in her arms and her leg felt heavy," he wrote. "The patient continues to complain of tingling in her left hand and weakness on her left side, [and] headache." The hospital records "grossly understated the impact on your life," Jim recalls, "because they couldn't see it."

A computed tomography (CT) scan of my brain that day showed swelling over the "right frontal area" and "some gas in the soft tissue," suggesting "a laceration of the frontal area of the scalp." Notes from Dr. Wheeler's physical examination describe me as "awake, lethargic." Dr. Wheeler attempted to give me an MRI to get a better look at my brain. But I was "unable to tolerate" the test, owing to "headache and noise." It apparently sounded to me like someone was pounding on a metal trash can inside my head.

The next three weeks brought "endless assessment," Jim recalls, a parade of occupational therapists, speech therapists, and cognitive therapists and neurologists, measuring my vital signs, my motor skills and reflexes, my diminished arm and leg strength, my ability to sit up without falling back over. A social worker was assigned as my care coordinator and she met regularly with other members of my care "team" to assess my progress and to develop a course of therapy.

"The right side of your face and the left side of your body were paralyzed to the point where you couldn't eat properly or sit in a chair," Jim recalls. "You couldn't feed yourself. You couldn't hold a spoon. Not that you even understood what a spoon was."

Jim says that I seemed overly sensitive to everything around me. Light, noise, movement—everything hurt. And I became upset every time I saw anybody enter my room. It was frustrating to the point of physical pain for me to try to tell a story again and again to each new nurse or therapist, when I had such a limited vocabulary and no real memory of what had happened.

Jim recalls spending most of the first week in the hospital. He felt profoundly protective of me and tried his damnedest to keep things around me quiet and calm. Jim asked if the hospital could have the same people assigned to my care every day. But every day, new nurses would arrive. They would turn all the lights up, and I would wince in pain.

"The frustrating thing was having to explain to every caregiver the whole story again and again,"

Jim recalls, "There was this presumption, looking at you, that you'd be able to do X, Y, and Z. And you simply couldn't. And then the doctors would get frustrated, the nurses would get frustrated, the therapists would get frustrated. You didn't understand."

Jim recalls the exact moment he realized the depth of my injury. At some point a nurse or therapist came with what looked like a toddler's board book that included nothing but colors and shapes. She sat with me and tested me: "Su, this is a red square. Turn the page. Su, what was on the previous page?" And I responded, "I don't know." Jim and the woman shared a look. "And that's the point when I realized just how whacked things were," Jim recalls.

My mother arrived on the evening of Tuesday, May 24. Jim met her at the airport. "We went out to supper," she recalls. "And then he took me to the garage to show me the fan that had fallen on your head. He said, 'This is what hit her.' And I said, 'Lord have mercy.' " Mom says she stayed until the weekend, mostly babysitting the boys so Jim could spend time at the hospital. She doesn't remember much of that visit. She recalls that "you had no idea who I was" when she first visited me in the hospital. But she also remembers the two of us carrying on conversations at my bedside. "I think what went through my mind when I saw you was, 'Well, Su has had this terrible accident, but she always bounces back from everything, and she's going to be okay.' "

May 25 was Jim's and my wedding anniversary. Barb, my eldest sister, customarily called me on that day. But this time, when she tried to call, "there was something wrong with the phone. The call wouldn't go through," Barb recalls. She kept trying, and then she tried again on the twenty-sixth. "And my mother answered the phone," Barb recalls. "And that was odd, because my parents and Jim didn't get along. They hadn't approved of the marriage. I probably said something like, 'Why are you there? Where's Su?' And she said that you were in the hospital." Mom told Barb there had been an accident, and that I had been in a coma and in the ICU.

"I was shocked and freaked out," Barb recalls. "And I remember thinking, 'Why had nobody told me in the first place?' " That night, Barb made a note in her journal: *Why??? Dear God, Please be with Su.*

Barb asked her boss for time off from work. They sat together in her office and prayed for me. Then, on Saturday, May 28, she and her husband, Scott, awoke at dawn and drove 850 miles from Urbana, Illinois, to Fort Worth. That evening, Jim took them to see me.

"We walked into the room, and it was you but you showed no signs of recognition of us," she recalled. "I will never, ever forget you looking at me and not knowing who I was. It was horrible. I said, 'I'm your sister, Barb.' And you said, 'Oh, okay,' like we were new people to you."

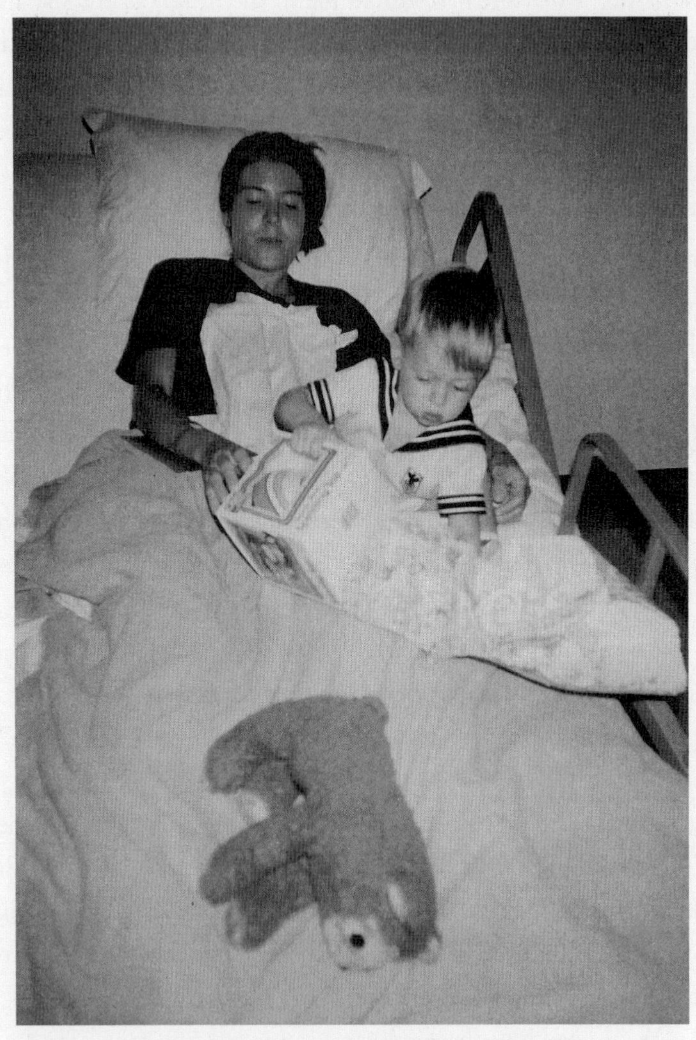

In the hospital after my injury with two-year-old Benjamin,
June 1988. The bear, Byron, is something Jim brought
from home in an attempt to trigger my memory.

The boys were making noise, and Barb says that I seemed overtaxed, as if "you didn't know how to deal with all of this input." The nurse brought in a meal tray, placed it in front of me, and left. Barb remembers that I, with my weakened left side, couldn't peel the Saran Wrap off of the containers by myself.

"You looked perfectly fine," Barb recalls. "You had about an inch-long cut on your forehead, and that's the only thing that looked different about you. It was just a little red stripe. There was no bandage. There was nothing, except for the vacant look in your eyes." My speech was slow. What I said was pretty low level. Very simple. Barb says I seemed to think that I *should* know who Jim and the kids were, but there wasn't that connection. There was nothing. "It was all very superficial and all very 'now' kind of talk, because there wasn't anything else. We were never in your room for more than an hour. We could tell that us being there, especially the boys being there . . . we could tell that that was just too overwhelming."

Barb recalls Jim's being hard on the hospital staff: "He's the kind of person who, if he feels like something's not going the way it should, he'll make his voice heard in an aggressive sort of way. I think there were times in the hospital when he expected things to go differently, and he made it very clear that he expected things to be different."

Jim's biggest complaint with the hospital staff was over the times I fell or slipped out of my chair. "You were always a very headstrong person. It's hard to know how many of your falls were just you taking risks," Barb says. "But I think Jim immediately blamed the staff for everything that wasn't perfect about your care." Meanwhile, in the hospital, the extent of the damage my brain had suffered was becoming clearer day by day as my hospital records show:

Tuesday, May 24

Before dawn, a nurse notes that I am "awake, responding well to orientation questions, much less lethargic, initiating conversation quite well." Later in the morning, another nurse notes that I am complaining of double vision and a headache that "never goes away."

A new neurologist, Dr. Guillermo Antonio Guzman, arrives and examines me. He writes, "I think with *positive* physical therapy/occupational therapy/speech input and support, she will improve over time. I've told her control of life cannot be complete but that she will have to [resume] activity anyway." He instructs someone to "try and get an objective idea" of my diminished strength on my left side. "Be positive; express doubts to me," he writes. He notes that I complain of a "constant, throbbing headache" as well as photophobia, nausea, and dizziness that comes whenever I sit up or swing my feet over the side of the bed. He also notes, "Memory short/long-term poor, but improving." Dr. Guzman recommends that I be assigned "memory exercises".

Wednesday, May 25

A rehabilitation doctor, Dr. Wilson Garcia, visits me. "Standing and sitting balance are poor," he notes. "She does not walk. She needs assistance with her ABCs." On the brighter side, I start to "control bladder and bowels."

An occupational therapist, Andrea Clark, assesses my ADL skills, or "activities of daily living": I "refused to sit up" because of dizziness and headaches. I require "a minimal assist" to eat, but I am able to brush my teeth unaided. I show short- and long-term memory problems in dealing with the world around me, and I have difficulty counting by twos. A neurological test finds me "unable to differentiate hot and cold, sharp from dull" on my left arm and leg.

Thursday, May 26

Dr. Garcia notes, "Patient is more alert today. She is talking more and smiling. She is progressing well," although "she is not walking yet."

Later in the day, Dr. Guzman seems to reach the opposite conclusion. "She may need more prolonged rehabilitation efforts than I originally thought," he writes, "and rehab floor is looking more necessary every day she doesn't achieve a minimal ADL status. Will discuss."

An occupational therapist gives me a series of tests. "Patient especially has problems with visual memory," the therapist writes, "but also appears to have problems with spatial orientation and visual discrimination," and my response time is "very slow."

A speech therapist describes me as "alert and cooperative" but notes "she rarely meets eye gaze, frequently averting eyes, particularly while forming responses to test questions." The therapist continues: "Patient has earned college degree in English. [What? Where did that come from?] She expressed frustration [about] feeling like a first grader in her responses." [I wonder if I actually said "first grader"] In one test I fail to remember any of three words a minute after they were shown to me. I also fail a test of judgment and reasoning. That afternoon, a nurse writes, "Patient asked to rate headache on a scale of 1–10, with 10 being the worst. Patient said headache was a 10."

Friday, May 27

A therapist writes that I "complain of dizziness," but I am able to sit for ten minutes without overwhelming nausea, which shows improvement. When the therapist gives me a brush, I am unable to use it on my hair. "She said it felt like the first time she had ever held a brush," the therapist writes. I am also unable to "demonstrate how to drink from a cup." The therapist concludes, "I suspect motor planning problems, or an inability to execute an unfamiliar sequence of movements."

Dr. Garcia notes the need to ask approval from our HMO for my admission to the hospital's rehab unit.

Monday, May 30

My pupils have returned to their proper size. I attempt to sit in a chair but become faint, and my blood pressure dips. I am helped back to bed.

A nurse, apparently new to my care, notes, "Light hurts eyes. Requests that it be turned off." A different nurse, also new, writes that I am "demanding," and that I require "frequent teaching and encouragement. Calls for nurse to raise and lower head of bed." The nurse seems not to connect my need for "teaching" to my memory loss.

Tuesday, May 31

The next day, I was transferred to the hospital's rehabilitation floor. In the rehab unit, there was much talk of therapy and goal setting. To cope with my memory problem, the leader of my treatment team told Jim, "Bring in things your wife would recognize." Jim brought in a boom box and some cassettes of music he thought I would remember: Pink Floyd, the Beatles, the Who, "classic rock things that you'd grown up on and loved." It appears that I enjoyed the music, but I didn't remember it. Later Jim was instructed to fetch my bicycle. My recovery had progressed to the point that the therapists wanted to work on my balance and bilateral movement. Two very large interns and I went up to the roof of the hospital, and I "rode" my bike, with the interns holding on either side to catch me if I fell. Somehow I had not forgotten how to pedal a bike.

"Even with the paralysis, you still had a lot of muscle tone," Jim recalled. "You were professional-athlete-grade fit. And your body seemed to have retained its sense of what was there. It was almost as if maybe the muscle memory wasn't completely affected by the accident. And once you could tap into that, you progressed. Quickly. You were released from the hospital in just a few weeks, not eight months like I had been originally told."

That's a rosy picture of how things went, but it may not be the whole story. Jim says that within a day of my relocation to the rehab floor, he arrived at my room and found me "in a heap on the floor." I had fallen out of my chair. "There were instructions. You weren't supposed to be left alone in a chair," Jim recalls. "You weren't supposed to be left alone at all when you were out of bed." Jim complained loudly about the mishap. His rising dissatisfaction with my care prompted several notations in the hospital records. Did this incident factor into the decision to send me home only a few days later?

After Barb and Scott left, Jim called my mom again. "He said, 'They've gone. I need help.' " Mom drove the five hours up from

Houston to Fort Worth again over Memorial Day weekend with Mark, my younger brother. Mark says he has no memory of this particular trip.

Jim, Mom, and Mark visited me in the rehabilitation wing. I still didn't recognize Mom; but she claims that I recognized Mark, the sibling to whom I had been perhaps closest in the years before I met Jim. "You didn't know me, you didn't know Jim, you didn't know the kids, but you seemed to know Mark when he came in," Mom recalls. I wonder if I had been told he was coming, or if recognizing Mark was one of those rare times when some freakish "gift" of a moment of meaning was given to me. Talk during that visit turned to my childhood, and suddenly some old memories of mine seemed to break through.

Mom says: "I remember talking to you and out of the blue you started talking about *Catcher in the Rye.* And I said, 'That's a book you read in high school.' You even remembered the name of the high school teacher that had assigned the book. And then just as quickly, it was gone."

My *Catcher in the Rye* moment was the first of just two instances in which I would reclaim memories from my old life, two fleeting glimpses of a lost past. Both would prove short-lived. "I thought, 'Oh, well, things are beginning to come back,' " Mom recalls. "I didn't realize that she would have these little instances where things would pop in and then be gone forever."

Much of my stay in the rehab unit followed a similar pattern: moments of seeming progress, followed by sudden relapses.

~

In the rehab admission papers, Dr. Garcia writes, "The patient has been confused and disoriented. She cannot walk. Her left side is weaker than her right side. She also complains of headaches." He notes, "Sitting balance is poor." He recommends physical, occupational, and speech therapy and states, "The patient will be in our head injury program."

Turning me over to the rehab team, Dr. Guzman later states that my condition has improved somewhat during my hospitalization but that "following 2–3 days of modest gains, she has plateaued." My "short-term memory is poor," he writes, "but this improved during her hospitalization and long-term memory seems fairly unaffected." I am "oriented to name, place, [and] date."

In summary, he writes, "Since she is young and the impact of her disability would be great on her family . . . it has been decided that an aggressive, acute rehabilitation stay is in order with as positive an attitude as possible to be generated for the patient."

Dr. Guzman notes, "plans for child care need to be made for a 4–6 week period to allow adequate physical therapy/occupational therapy trial."

Someone types a modest checklist of goals for my therapy: sitting and standing balance; wheelchair mobility; gait; communication skills; swallowing. Another writer notes that I might benefit from "dim-lit room, low noise, calm environment."

I am told to keep a logbook to aid my memory. Can I read? Can I write? I am assigned a case manager, Penny Perry. Penny meets with Jim. After the meeting, she notes, "Husband would like to be very involved in wife's rehab program."

Wednesday, June 1

In the morning, I have some sort of breakdown, triggered, perhaps, by awakening in an unfamiliar room, or by Jim's return to work and resulting absence from my bedside. Penny Perry, the case manager, notes: "[Jim] initially expressed concern that his return to work caused her agitation. Mr. Meck also, somewhat hesitantly, expressed concern for financial needs and his need to return to work, but [he is] concerned that he should be with his wife. Reassured often that Mrs. Meck is well cared for, and probably environmental change, i.e., move to new room, new faces, change in routine caused rise in agitation. After Mrs. Meck regained her composure, we discussed uses of her journal as a communication device."

A psychologist meets with me and Jim. He notes, "Patient was acutely distressed because husband was not here this A.M. . . . Patient extremely dependent on husband and expressing 'I don't understand.' Obviously she is having marked difficulty comprehending emotionally charged and abstract information. It will probably help to limit [the] number of different staff working with patient. Familiarity with fewer staff would probably increase rapport and cooperation and reduce agitation and resistance."

Someone notes that Jim has requested "something other than what was served on menu for patient at lunch. He said the transfer to rehab unit has made patient very disoriented and confused, therefore she was not able to eat."

Paula McMillen, a medical social worker, takes a psychosocial assessment of me. Both Jim and I are interviewed, but I am "medicated and somewhat confused," so most of the narrative comes from Jim.

McMillen states, "Patient has a mother with whom she does not have a good relationship, an older sister from Illinois who is presently here visiting, a brother in Ohio, and a sister in Virginia." She also refers to a nonexistent "youngest sister," whom Jim describes as "lost." Where did the story of this lost sister come from? Did Jim invent her for some reason? Or was this just another case of patient mix-up and medical record confusion? It's discrepancies like this one that leave me struggling with feelings of fear and frustration about my care in the hospital.

A nurse notes that I have begun making entries in my journal to help my memory. I would give anything to see what I was able to "write" in my supposed "journal." My cynical theory is that there was no writing, and no journal, but because there was something in my chart (or somebody's chart) about it, the nurse felt the need to comment on my progress and keep this dream alive. Jim does remember some sort of a "word book" that was kept for me, but he doesn't remember exactly how it was maintained. However, he thinks it was highly unlikely that I personally wrote down anything of substance while in the hospital. He vaguely remembers my practicing writing out my name on large pieces of handwriting paper, as well as reading a few pages of Dr. Seuss's *Hop on Pop* out loud to him a day or two before being released.

Thursday, June 2

Dr. Guzman suggests "that there is a nonorganic"—i.e., psychological component—"to patient's complaints," and that "psychological support is our single best approach to maximal improvement."

This notation marks one of the first references to the doctors' growing frustration—if not outright doubt—about my condition, a source of unending upset and stress for me for years to come.

Jim and I somehow celebrate Benjamin's second birthday in

my room. A nurse notes: "Quiet birthday party for 2-year-old son OK'd in patient's room. Sits for no longer than half hour." Doctors and therapists list many short-term goals for me:

Dressing with minimal assistance
Carry-over of instructions and knowledge from A.M. to P.M.
Have patient maintain sitting balance for over five minutes
Increase memory for daily activities
Improve verbal expression
Decrease agitation

Friday, June 3

A physical therapist notes, "Patient stated she feels like she is falling when she is sitting up." I work on my sitting balance. The therapist notes, "balance zero."

Dr. Garcia notes I am taking medication "for agitation."

Monday, June 6

I tell a therapist I fell out of my chair two days earlier, on Saturday. The therapist says I tell her: "She decided she had to start working harder on her problems."

The therapist makes another checklist of activities for me to work on:

Tandem walking [with an aide]
Braiding
Walking on toes
Showering

I complete a "bike evaluation" and a "jazzercise activity."

Jim and I meet again with Paula McMillen, the medical social worker. She notes, "Patient has made remarkable progress since last week—is walking, and has shown significant improvement in memory, coordination, etc." She also hints that Jim is growing impatient: "Mr. Meck insisted on accelerated therapy based on her exceptional progress over the weekend." She approves an evening pass for the following night, probably for Jim and me to have dinner together at home. I have begun recreational therapy on my bicycle and occupational therapy in the kitchen. The social worker notes, "Patient and husband very eager for discharge by end of week."

A nurse notes "reassessment of reading and cognitive skills due to significant change in patient's status over the weekend. Both areas [now] appear to be functional." Was this perhaps the day when I was practicing writing my name and reading *Hop on Pop*?

Tuesday, June 7

I tell a therapist "I am feeling good today." However, she notices and writes that my "patience with everyday activities is very short."

More testing. More results: "Patient manifested mild word-finding difficulties as well as mild to moderate mental calculation difficulties." The psychologist, David Wilson, prepares another checklist:

Attention: severely impaired
Language comprehension: severely impaired
Memory: moderately impaired
Calculation: moderately impaired
Abstract reasoning and judgment: severely impaired

A nurse notes, "Patient very angry and agitated at times by external stimuli. Patient and husband require teaching re safety, limitations, medications."

Wednesday, June 8

Hospital notes suggest that Jim and I spent the previous evening home with family. A therapist writes, "Patient stated she became frustrated at home last night, too many people in the room."

I take (and apparently pass) a "safety evaluation": crossing a street, walking in a crowd, and riding a bike. On the bike evaluation, I start and stop on command and weave left and right to avoid objects tossed in front of me.

Thursday, June 9

Overnight, my condition seems to have improved dramatically. A chorus of upbeat reports signals my rapid recovery. My discharge is scheduled for the following day. A therapist notes, "Patient has shown remarkable improvement in all areas . . . Previous cognitive deficits appear resolved." Another therapist concurs: "Patient showed a dramatic change in status over the weekend [an odd statement, coming on a Thursday] and upon reassessment, all skills appear to be within normal limits, certainly functional for her to return home."

Dr. Garcia adds, "Patient is not agitated anymore."

My social worker notes, "Patient has met almost all her goals in a very short time, but still may have some mild cognitive deficits. [Personality tests] showed a lot of denial, probably related to head injury." For outpatient follow-up: "No therapies recommended, but psychotherapy is recommended."

Friday, June 10

"Home today," Dr. Garcia notes. "Patient and husband instructed about safety precautions. Dr. Wilson, the psychologist, meets with Jim and me to discuss "the benefits of supportive therapy. They declined, but said they would call if they felt the need. They [probably Jim] indicated that counseling was not a 'drug' that worked with them."

Another battery of tests. I am given the Wechsler Adult Intelligence Scale test and show an IQ of exactly 100 in the final write-up. Although buried in the middle of the report, is another reference that put my IQ at 70. On a test of visual-spatial skills, I perform at the level of a six-year-old. And on a personality test, I respond "in a defensive manner, attempting to present herself in the best possible light."

The psychologist notes my emotional fragility: "She has resources available to handle personal stresses of everyday living, but probably not the aftermath of a closed-head injury. She has strong need for affection and a tendency toward ill-considered, impulsive behavior. There are definite visual motor deficits which are exacerbated by her impulsivity." He concludes, "Patient and family's decision to not accept outpatient services is a negative prognosticator with regard to her overall recovery."

A nurse restates that my condition has improved "significantly" since the previous weekend. At this time my "cognitive and communication status are functional enough to return home." She writes, "No further speech or cognitive therapy [is] recommended on an outpatient basis." The nurse notes that I tell her I will have a nanny to help with the children at home.

Dr. Wilson Garcia writes an upbeat dismissal summary: "On admission to the rehabilitation unit, the patient could not walk and needed assistance with all of her activities of daily living. She was complaining of double vision and photophobic. The patient was started in our head injury program. She made a remarkable improvement to the point that when she left the hospital, she was walking by herself and doing all of her activities without any assistance. On admission to the rehabilitation unit, she was at cognitive level 4, and when she left she was at cognitive level 8." (Dr. Garcia is referring to the Rancho Levels of Cognitive Functioning Scale, used to assess patients who emerge from coma. A score of I is comatose. A 4 is "confused/agitated." An 8 is normal.) "This patient made a remarkable improvement," Dr. Garcia writes, although she was "agitated [sic] and she needed medication for that." Thus improved, he wrote, "the patient went back home with recommendations for outpatient psychotherapy."

And just like that, I was on my way home.

3

~

I Don't Remember

—Peter Gabriel

According to Miller family lore, I took a trip to Niagara Falls with my family when I was three. Walking along the rim, I heard the falls roaring in my ears and felt the mist pelting my face. Since I was so young, my parents didn't yet know just how bad my eyesight was. I could feel the mist and hear the roar, but couldn't see where those things were coming from. I grew frightened, and that fear swelled into panic. Suddenly I broke away from my mother's grip and dashed out into the street. Luckily, my parents grabbed me and pulled me out of the road before I could be hurt.

That episode, a visceral combination of sight, sound, and powerful emotion, is part of the shared heritage that binds the

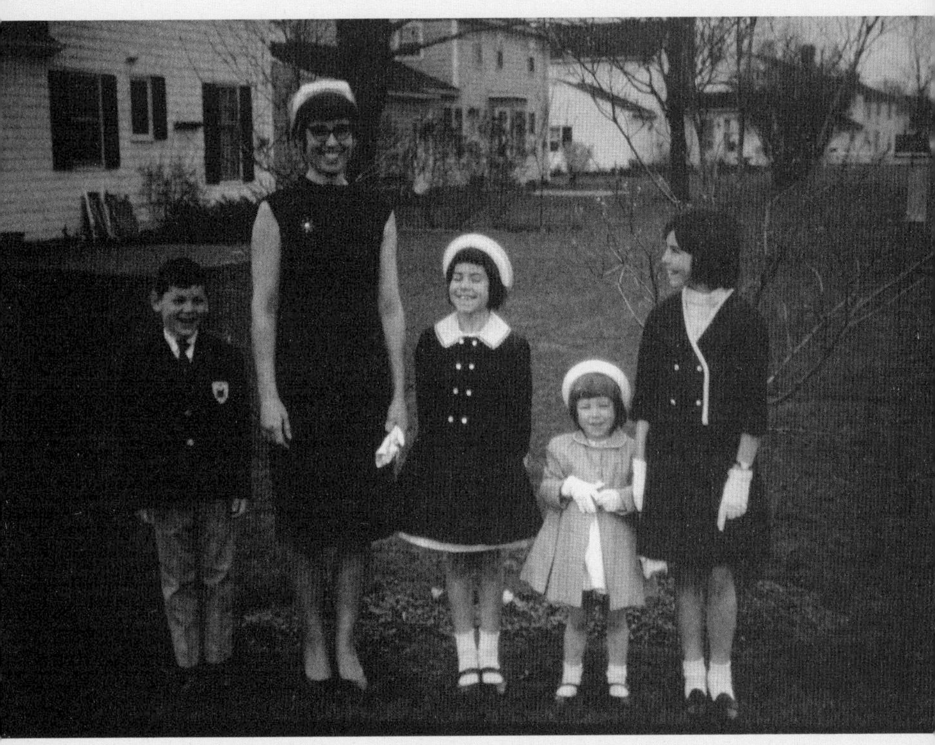

Left to right: my brother Rob, Mom, my sister Diane, me, and my sister Barb, Mentor, Ohio, Easter 1968

members of the Miller family—my family—together. It endures as a rich, nearly palpable memory within the minds of both Miller parents and each of their children, remote in time and space but instantly accessible to any Miller at the mere utterance of a simple prompt: *Remember when Su ran out into the street at Niagara Falls?*

Brain scientists call these "episodic memories"—recollections of specific events from one's lived experience. Episodic memory is thought to be a distinctly human trait, one of the few things that set us apart from the other animals, and perhaps the most important quality that defines each of us as individuals.

But I have no memory of that episode at Niagara Falls. In fact, I have no lingering episodic memory, not a stitch, from the first twenty-two years of my life. My sense of who I am, and my relationship with the other Millers, is entirely based on the events of the last twenty years.

≈

For most people, episodic memory is synonymous with memory itself. But it is only one of at least three different kinds of memory, along with "semantic memory" and "procedural memory." Each has a different purpose, and each resides in different places within the human brain.

Procedural memory is the remembered ability to perform tasks. We never forget how to ride a bike (or to walk, or to talk, or to swing a bat) because of the fundamental strength of our procedural memories. Semantic memory is the recollection of facts: names, concepts, and even specific events, but not events we recall as scenes from our own life. Most people have semantic memories of Woodstock; those who attended have episodic memories as well. All of my memories from childhood are semantic memories;

stories that have been told to me and stories that I can recite, but that don't feel like any real experiences I have lived. Anyone who has studied psychology in school will also remember the concept of short-term and long-term memories. Short-term memories are disposable, lasting only seconds or minutes: Post-its from our brain. We use short-term memory to recall the digits of a telephone number to be dialed once, the location of a coconut we just spotted in a tree, and other facts useful for our immediate survival but trivial in the broader course of life. Long-term memory is reserved for information useful beyond the present moment: the directions to our house; the phone numbers of loved ones; our blood type; our first date with a spouse.

Repetition—learning—consolidates short-term memories into long-term ones. The consolidation process can be voluntary, as in studying for an exam, or involuntary, as in those conditioning experiments with animals that used electric shocks and treats to "teach" the rat to find the pellet. Long-term memories can endure for weeks or years or decades. The human brain is forever sifting through memories, preserving the ones that matter for our survival and discarding those that don't. Memories are Darwinian: only the ones the brain deems most vital to our survival will, themselves, survive.

That was news to me. Jim remembers a dog-walk conversation that we had less than ten years ago when he first realized how I thought my memory was supposed to work. For most of my life I thought that other adults remembered every fact, every image, every scene they had ever lived, recording memories like a twenty-four-hour security camera. But I guess it makes sense: Who could possibly handle that much memory?

Our brain's anatomy plays a role in memory; the recall of a

memory is thought to involve several areas of the brain. Different regions record sights and sounds, numbers and names, motor skills and three-dimensional spaces. To recall a whole memory, the medial temporal lobe, a section at the brain's inner core, must fetch each individual component from different places in the brain. The medial temporal lobe is also thought to help us consolidate short-term episodic and semantic memories into long-term ones, although it does not control formation of procedural memories. The frontal lobe, behind the forehead, seems to help us understand episodic memories by helping the brain place them in context, so that they make sense as a coherent whole. Without a functioning frontal lobe, we might remember the Air and Space Museum as semantic, factual knowledge but forget the childhood visit that is the source of that memory.

Most people who suffer amnesia through injury, such as a football tackle or car accident, forget the things that happened shortly before the traumatic event, a mild form of what is called "retrograde" amnesia. The presumed reason is that the injury disrupts the memory-making process, erasing short-term memories before they can become long-term ones. Thus, a driver who hits a tree might never remember whatever he was doing or thinking in the minutes before the impact, because the collision interrupted the conversion of those items into enduring memories. In more serious cases, such as people with profound dementia or Alzheimer's disease, the oldest memories tend to be the safest. This is called Ribot's law, after the nineteenth-century French psychologist who first described this pattern. The destruction of memory "advances progressively from the unstable to the stable," from new memories to old, Ribot wrote.

Even people with severe cases of retrograde amnesia typically remember their earliest memories. But not everyone. Daniel Schacter, a Harvard psychologist, studied a man named Gene who, following a motorcycle accident, was "unable to recall a single specific episode from any time in his life." Gene suffered damage to both his frontal and temporal lobes. He can neither create new memories nor retrieve old ones. His brain does not obey Ribot's law.

Of all the amnesia victims studied by scientists, Gene's case may be the most like mine. I have what is called "complete retrograde amnesia." The injury knocked out not just my episodic memory but also most of my semantic memory, my knowledge of the world. According to Jim after the injury, my factual knowledge base was effectively empty: I didn't know who I was, and couldn't recall that I had a husband or children or the identities of my parents or siblings. I didn't know what a house was, or that I lived in one. I didn't know the purpose of school, or that I had ever attended one. I didn't know what a city was; the name *Fort Worth* did not register, nor did the terms *Texas, United States,* and *Earth.* I didn't know what a president was, and the name Ronald Reagan held no special significance for me.

I could speak, but my vocabulary extended to only maybe one hundred words. Jim tells me I couldn't recall the names of the objects around me—the clock, the bed, the door—or their functions. I didn't know what a utensil was, or how to use one. "And even after you figured out how to use a fork," Jim recalls, "you gripped it in a fist, like a toddler."

My hospital records offer some corroboration of Jim's memories. Nurses' logs show I struggled to answer simple "orientation" questions at times, although at other times (according to the medical records) I appear to have correctly stated who I was, where I was, and what day it was. It is possible I somehow bluffed my way through these questions, or maybe the nurses weren't paying very close attention to my answers. I certainly got through much of my life after the hospital through a combination of those two things.

For a long time after the accident, I suffered not just retrograde amnesia but also "anterograde amnesia," the inability to form new memories. For months (even years) afterward, I would wake up "lost" in unfamiliar places. According to Jim, I could carry on conversations with nurses and family in the hospital, but I would lose my train of thought after a few minutes, and I could manage such a conversation "only if the person stayed in sight." Communicating was a chore. "I remember [that] a lot—I would say a majority—of our communication became nonverbal, gesture-based," Jim recalls. "That said, I also recall a 'word book,' a spiral notebook one of your therapists helped you develop. She would drill you on the words and add a new word or two every day. I remember your excitement at recognizing a new word as new, and then writing it down. I remember it was an almost terrifyingly small list in the beginning, and being reassured by the therapist that it would get better, so much so that your learning and vocabulary would hit a critical mass, and your vocabulary growth would take off. It did. But I also remember you writing simple letters to family and asking for your word book to help you."

Here is a passage from a letter I wrote to my mother, shortly after the injury:

I hav to go to mor doctors be case fall lots to hitig head bad head ackes.

Like many other amnesiacs, I was lucky enough to retain some procedural memory. I didn't completely lose the ability to speak,

Dear Gramma and Grampa,
I got your letter today
Thankyou for riting. Maybe
not peple rite for me but I
rite letters to lots of peple
maybe Jim can rede letter
wen comes home for work later
Canot rede vary good I canot
we have film at store for
pictors I sendig. One for
Patrick crawlrg one for me
and Benjamin (look close)
or big slid in park for bike
ridig. long way to clime
up but good slid down.
Sorry canot come for
Patricks birth day prty
He will be one yers old.

This is one example of a letter I wrote to my grandparents about six months after my head injury.

although my vocabulary was severely limited. I didn't entirely forget how to sit, stand, or walk, although the partial paralysis on my left side made all those tasks much more difficult. Based on the story about my riding a bicycle on the hospital roof—albeit with help from two burly orderlies—it's clear that I must have been relatively strong and in good physical condition, which in turn may have helped with my overall recovery.

Other physical skills were lost. For instance, one nurse noted that I was unable to brush my hair, I was unable to drink from a cup, and I had to relearn how to eat. But as would later be the case for me socially, I proved particularly adept at mimicking the actions of others. A physical therapist discovered that I could accomplish some physical tasks while watching myself in a mirror (tasks that were beyond me without it), apparently tapping some deep muscle memory.

Like many amnesiacs, I am told I had trouble remembering that I even had a damaged memory. In the early days of my recovery, "you didn't seem to know that memory was an issue," Jim recalls, and I had to be frequently reminded of my deficits. "There were times when I had the sense that you knew something was terribly wrong, but that was generally, and perhaps exclusively, when you were being asked to do something that you couldn't do, or didn't understand what was being asked of you because you didn't understand the words being used."

≈

I have been told that my case is puzzling to scientists. The scope of my memory loss places me among the most severe cases of retrograde amnesia on record. Very few amnesiacs have lost all trace of episodic memory; very few are unable to recall a single life experience. I am unusual too in the extent of my recovery. But the most confounding part of my story, for scientists, is the lack of visible damage to my brain. I sustained a head injury; of that there is no doubt. But the doctors who examined me after the accident found only faint evidence of palpable injury to my brain itself: on the CT scan I had in the hospital, and on an MRI of my spine that showed a sharply diminished flow of blood in the right vertebral artery, consistent with the partial paralysis on my left side. Those findings are, to this day, the sole direct evidence of physical damage to my brain.

"We always try to relate these conditions to neuroanatomy": in other words, to trace memory loss to damage in specific areas of the brain," says Larry Squire, a memory scientist at the University of California, San Diego. "And we know what kinds of damage cause what types of conditions. But the cases that are particularly hard to relate to anatomy are head injuries," because those injuries are random and unpredictable, and the exact location of damage can be hard to pinpoint.

According to Daniel Schacter, the Harvard scientist who studied the amnesiac Gene, damage to the medial temporal region at the inner core of my brain might have compromised my ability to form new episodic and semantic memories, and such damage might also have hindered my recall of old memories. Damage to the frontal lobe as recorded in my CT scan would affect my ability to comprehend the source of episodic memory "scenes," and my capacity to be aware of my memory loss.

But because my episodic memory was completely erased, Schacter says, "You would expect to see more evidence of brain damage" than my brain scans revealed. "It doesn't sound like there was a detectable brain lesion."

However, Michael Yassa, a researcher at Johns Hopkins, points out that MRI technology has improved dramatically since the 1980s. He thinks it's possible that if I got an MRI today, doctors would see some damage that wouldn't have been visible back then. Assuming that I did, in fact, suffer an injury to my brain, there are at least three possibilities for where the damage could lie, according to Yassa. "One is, it could be a frontal lobe problem," the area of the brain related to managing and making sense of episodic memories. "Two, it could be a hippocampus problem"; the hippocampus is an organ in the inner core of the brain that is critical to forming new episodic and semantic memories and to creating permanent memories. "Three, it could be a problem with the connection between the two." If brain imaging shows no serious damage to either region, Yassa reasons, then the problem likely lies in that connection.

Larry Squire, at San Diego, says my case is particularly unusual in that I suffered "such extensive retrograde amnesia and not so much anterograde amnesia, at least not much that has persisted." Amnesics with severe loss of past memories tend to also have chronic trouble making new memories. Squire suggests that I might have suffered damage to the lateral temporal cortex, the area adjacent to the medial temporal region and associated with long-term memory storage, in contrast to the medial temporal "core," where those memories are built. "If one had a lesion that was primarily in the lateral temporal cortex, but the damage was such that it was still possible" for brain signals "to get into the medial temporal lobe," such an injury "could approximate what's being described," he says.

All of these scientists are quick to note that complete retrograde amnesia is very rare—so rare that it is sometimes called

"Hollywood amnesia," existing more in movies than in real life. Yassa believes the reason for my total memory loss could be that I was relatively young at the time of my injury. He says it is possible that, at the age of twenty-two, none of my memories were fully consolidated and etched into permanent storage. Many amnesia patients are much older than twenty-two when their memory deficits appear, and their earliest memories are, at that point, several decades in the past. And scientists don't know precisely how long it takes the brain to fully consolidate memories, to render them permanent. It's thought to take years, at least, and possibly decades. By Yassa's theory, my life memories might have been in a transitory state at the time of my injury: not in the memory bank, so to speak, but in the truck, on its way to the bank. The injury robbed the truck. If that's the case, my memories are not buried somewhere within my brain, waiting for some hypnotist or surgeon to access them: they are gone. Schacter, the Harvard scientist, disagrees: at age twenty-two, he reasons, my early childhood memories would have been fully consolidated into permanent storage. That I cannot access them is exceedingly unusual, he says, but not unprecedented; remember Gene, who lost all of his life memories at thirty.

⁓

There is one other possibility, one that has always haunted me: the possibility that my memory loss could be psychological. "Functional," or "psychogenic amnesia" is memory loss caused not by brain injury or illness but by some psychological reason. The classic Hollywood case is the Hitchcock film *Spellbound*: A young doctor, played by Gregory Peck, has forgotten who he is and taken on another man's identity. A glamorous therapist, Ingrid Bergman, helps him reclaim his identity by escorting him back to the place where he lost it: a mountain precipice where a friend had fallen to his death. Revisiting the site, the doctor relives the memory, and his lost identity comes flooding back.

After my release from the hospital, Jim took me to the neurologist about every two weeks. Jim says we lived for these appointments. One day, we showed up late, and were crushed when he refused to see me. At the same time, the way Jim tells it, I get the feeling that these appointments were an exercise in futility. The doctor would insist on seeing me alone, and afterward, I would have no idea of what I had said to him, or what he said to me. Then the doctor would give Jim a ninety-second generic summary and conclude with something like, "I'm not seeing any change." He could find no physiological explanation for my memory loss, or for the lingering numbness in my left hand and foot. He gave me another MRI, and when the results came back he told Jim, "I see absolutely nothing here. Her brain looks completely normal. I see no damage." And then under his breath, "I think she's just making all this up."

Jim stopped taking me to the neurologist.

I get the feeling from everything I have heard that the doctors and everyone else in the medical community were maybe just as frustrated as Jim and I were. There didn't seem to be any test or imaging that explained my symptoms. Everybody had told Jim that all of this was going to just be temporary, and when it wasn't, it somehow became my fault. I was faking it. It was all in my head, psychological. And that makes absolutely no sense to me at all! Why would I *want* to be this way? Why would I—why would anyone—*choose* to be this way?

Happily for me, though, the facts don't seem to bear out the possibility that it is "all in my head." Psychogenic amnesia is "much rarer than amnesia that results from brain damage and easy to distinguish from it," according to Larry Squire. When amnesia is psychological in origin, the damage is typically limited to past memories; the ability to form new memories is not impaired. People with psychogenic amnesia sometimes lose episodic memories of their own lives but retain semantic memories about the world. Others lose both episodic and semantic memories. Psychogenic amnesia can block the memory of a single event, a full life chapter, or a person's entire past history. Often, psychogenic amnesia clears up in a relatively short span, and lost memories are recovered.

Squire and colleagues carried out the first study of a large group of patients with psychogenic amnesia, ten cases in all. The researchers found that almost no one in the group had trouble forming new memories. But eight of the ten had retrograde amnesia that lingered for more than a year after its onset.

Squire's research found that the circumstances of each case varied according to how each patient "thinks amnesia works," because their brains created the problem. So they forgot the things that they thought amnesiacs should forget, and they remembered the things they thought amnesia patients should remember. For some patients, the amnesia itself was triggered "by an incident that people believe should cause a memory problem," such as a car wreck or a blow on the head, Squire says.

The range of symptoms in psychogenic amnesia is "as variable as humankind's concept of what memory is and how it works," Squire and his coauthors wrote. In one recent case, a Florida amnesiac awoke each day having forgotten all that she had experienced in the previous day. The case was unique, and researchers concluded her amnesia was constructed to precisely replicate the memory loss depicted in the film *50 First Dates.* That film became her template for how amnesia works. The patient later improved in therapy.

People often wonder why Jim and I didn't have more interest in my condition, and why we didn't seek more help from neurologists or psychiatrists in rebuilding my life. I have certainly thought about this question a lot recently. Jim and I have discussed at length why we eventually gave up on the medical community. The easy and perhaps blunt answer is: frustration. My frustration. Jim's frustration. The frustration of the many and varied doctors and other professionals. Multiple tests were given. Many images were taken. They always seemed to come back "inconclusive." There was no pill to give me. There was no surgery to perform. Therefore, it must just be in my head.

I think it is also relevant to mention here that I didn't actually think there was anything wrong with me. I didn't get that I had any memory issues or problems with speech and understanding. I didn't know that I was different in any way from anyone else until many, many years later. Jim noticed a lot of my difficulties. I was slow in speech. I repeated myself a great deal. I was forgetful and often got lost. I didn't read anymore. But because I, for the most part, outwardly seemed okay to him most of the time, he tended to ignore the countless little things. He just wanted me to be okay so we could move on with our lives.

I was twenty-three and Jim was twenty-five. We had two young boys who were a bit rambunctious, a bit disheveled, and who also

4

~

You Can't Always Get What You Want

—Rolling Stones

After being in the hospital for only three weeks, I was released to go home. That in itself was a small miracle, because Jim was initially told that with injuries such as mine, it wasn't unusual for people to stay hospitalized for eight months, maybe longer. But medically speaking, my MRI scans did not show the doctors any kind of persistent or residual damage to my brain. So in their opinion, I was all better. In the words of those Bible-thumping evangelical preachers, "I was *healed!*"

The rehabilitation staff told Jim, "Our goal is to get someone who is five to fifteen percent functional to twenty to thirty percent." I was quite possibly at 70 or 80 percent. I was the god-damned valedictorian of head injury patients! The head physician on the ward told Jim, "I'm not sure there is much more we can do for Su. She could be here another six months, and I don't know if her condition would change all that much." Jim thinks that my relatively young age combined with my health and level of athleticism at the time had a lot to do with my comparatively short and rather miraculous "recovery" and early release.

~

The hospital records present my release as if it was a matter of mutual agreement. That is how Jim remembers it. But in hindsight, my discharge seems rather abrupt, certainly considering that three days earlier, a neuropsychologist had described me as moderately to severely impaired in five major cognitive areas.

"I remember Jim kept saying, 'We've got to get her out of the hospital, because they keep dropping her on her head,' " Barb recalls.

My mom: "I do think you should have been in the hospital longer than you were."

Here are a few of my own thoughts about all of this now: Jim was driving everyone crazy at the hospital with his demands and interference. Jim didn't know what to do with Benjamin and Patrick. He had to go to work, and he had run out of, or used up, all his options for babysitting (i.e., friends and family). I think I was somehow "fast-tracked" out of the hospital, either because of Jim's behavior or our medical insurance coverage. All of a sudden, people started writing in my chart, that my problem was most likely something psychological rather than physical and I was shown the door.

My sister Barb is convinced that it was too early for me to go home. To this day she tells me, "You were not ready. You should have gone to a rehab facility, or you should have gone home with a crew of therapists; someone to help you with speech, a physical therapist to help with gross motor skills, and an occupational therapist to help with fine motor tasks. You couldn't write. Walking and moving around was hard for you. You couldn't even use your left side, and you were left-handed! And you had two little kids." Barb never thought it was a good idea for me to go home when I did, but as she tells it, "I couldn't do anything about it. And you couldn't do anything about it. You didn't know anything. I couldn't really talk to Jim. He wasn't there to listen."

Let's think about this for a second, shall we? And part of this will just be me speculating, of course. Did I know who I was? After three weeks in the hospital? I probably knew my name was Su Meck. Did I know Jim, Benjamin, and Patrick? Did I understand *husband? Marriage? Son? Brother? Mother? Father?* Did I make connections as to who these people were in relationship to me? My guess is no, I didn't. I probably didn't have a clue as to how to take care of myself, let alone two very young boys. Was going home to a house I didn't know, with a family that might just as well have been assigned to me, really a safe, smart, logical next step? Looking back, I don't think it was safe, smart, or logical. And yet, that is exactly what happened.

I may never know why. Maybe Jim didn't have a choice. Maybe it was some kind of insurance decision. If the insurance company decided that I was well enough, they would put pressure on the doctors to have me released. Jim certainly would not have been able to pay my medical expenses without insurance. Was Jim ever told what services may have been available to me once I was home? He tells me he doesn't remember anything like that ever being dis-

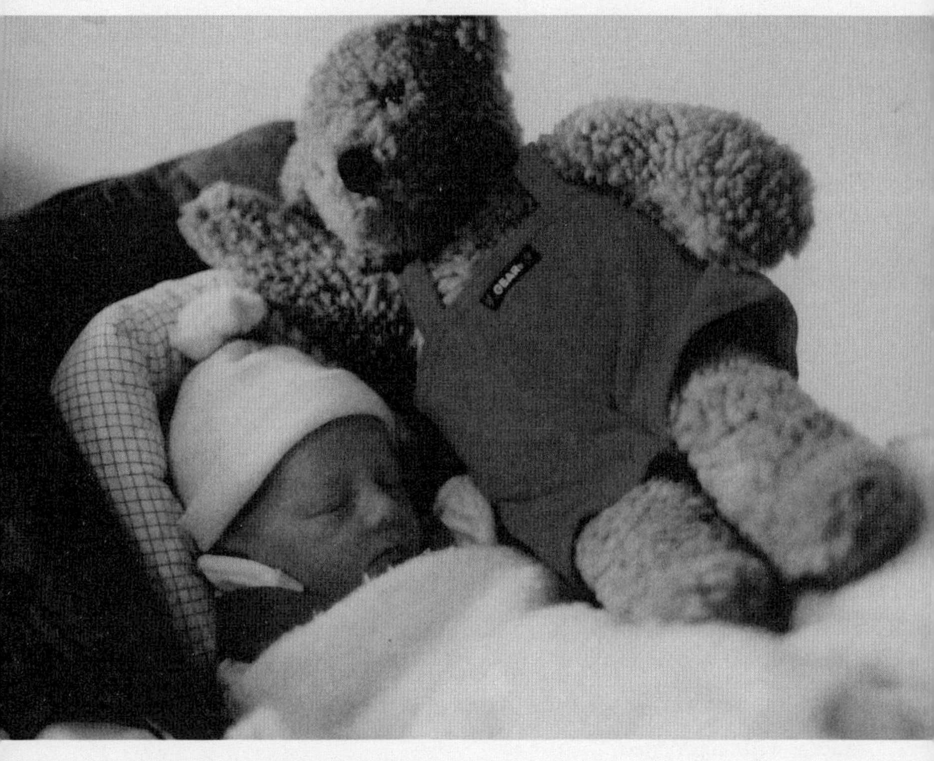

The photo of Patrick reaching the magic five-pound weight so he could leave the hospital. This hung in the hallway of our home on El Greco.

cussed. I find myself wondering, Why didn't Jim ask? But I have to keep telling myself, all of this was happening and all of these decisions were being made when Jim was just twenty-four years old.

~

Whatever the reason, I was released from the hospital and taken to live in a house I did not remember. The 1970s gold-flecked linoleum and shag carpeting, the green scratchy couch, the brown kitchen cupboards, the large backyard surrounded by a privacy fence. None of these things registered with me. Jim remembers me walking hesitantly down the hallway that led from the family room back to the bedrooms. He recalls me just staring at all of the family photographs that were hanging there. "That's me!" I said, pointing to my image. "And that's me, too!" I recognized myself in the more recent photographs, but I had no recollection of the places where even a single one of the pictures had been taken, or any of the stories behind them. I was not able to identify any of the other people—other friends and family—in the photos. It was sort of like being airbrushed into a life. A real-life *Twilight Zone.*

I walked into the kitchen and opened every single cupboard and drawer. There was nothing recognizable about any of this stuff. I probably didn't even know what most of the items were called, or what they could possibly be used for. The hospital was all I knew. Everything in this house was unfamiliar, and I can only imagine how bewildering and daunting that unfamiliarity would have been to me. What would it have felt like for me to not know even the names of objects in my own home? But then I think, did I even care? Did I ask questions, or was I just too overwhelmed? Jim doesn't really remember much of my first days at home. I'm thinking having me there again was just as weird for him as it was for me.

He does remember my first "lightning strike," though. It occurred that very first night home. Jim thinks I was trying to help him make dinner. (Maybe I should have just stayed out of that kitchen).

I don't remember this, but after my accident, when I was still in the hospital, one of the things I was taught how to do was make tuna fish salad. I am sure tuna fish salad was used as a "training food" for food preparation and kitchen safety purposes because there are a lot of different steps in preparing tuna fish, as well as a lot of learning how to use kitchen tools. I was taught (over the course of several days) everything from operating a can opener, to properly and safely using a sharp knife and cutting board, to using a measuring cup, to stirring all the ingredients together with a spoon in a big bowl, and then to finally manipulating another (not sharp) knife in order to spread the tuna fish on bread. I was taught how to properly wash and peel fruits and vegetables, and even how to boil an egg in a pot of water on the stove.

Armed with this vast expanse of knowledge, I was sent home with the expectation that I would be able to feed my family and myself.

And that is exactly what I did. I fed my family tuna fish. Breakfast. Lunch. Dinner. Did anyone complain? I don't know. Did Jim give the boys other stuff to eat? Did he make himself other stuff to eat? Again, I don't know. Did I attempt to cook or prepare anything else? I seriously doubt it. I had been told that "tuna fish equals meal, and meal is what you eat."

But on my very first night home, dinner was probably something really simple for Jim to prepare, like frozen chicken nuggets and french fries that he could just throw onto a cookie sheet and toss into the oven. But the cooking noises of clattering pans and utensils, the bright overhead kitchen light, the commotion of two small, excited, and hungry children was all too much, and I was suddenly slumped on the floor. Jim saw me fall; saw me on the floor motionless in the area between the kitchen and the garage. My eyes were open, but I was unresponsive to his voice. It was "almost as if a light switch had been turned off," he recollects. This very same thing had happened a few times in the hospital, but apparently not frequently enough for anybody to be concerned. (And once again I think, Really? Hmm!) After maybe five minutes on the kitchen floor, a very long five minutes, I slowly became aware of my surroundings, and I pulled myself up. Enter: Piercing Headache and Foggy Confusion! When there is "lightning," "Piercing Headache" and "Foggy Confusion" always follow. All three (Lightning, Headache, Foggy Confusion) are to me, even to this day, actual characters or creatures with definite identities of their own, living in my brain somehow. Not in a "I hear voices in my head" kind of way, but instead in sort of a construction-crew kind of way. When lightning comes, that precise kind of headache and that certain kind of foggy confusion will always follow. They are a three-pronged team that works together in my brain. Doing what? I don't know. And because I was never able to describe it competently enough to doctors or other medical professionals without sounding like a crazy person, these three entities continue to be in my life even now.

Back then, I think, a broader realization was beginning to sink in for Jim: I wasn't "getting" any of this. For example, we would take walks as a family around the neighborhood, to the post office, or to the park, and I continued to not have any idea where I was or where I was going. I wouldn't remember walking along the exact same sidewalk, even if I had walked the route earlier in the week, or earlier that same day. I was lost in my own suburban neighborhood. But if Jim was even aware of this, he surely didn't know what to do about it.

My lightning strikes continued, with a frequency of one every two or three days. Jim just thought they were caused by some sort of sensory overload that would overwhelm my nervous system, which in turn would trigger a shutdown. Almost as if I had blown a fuse, I would collapse and be unresponsive for several minutes.

~

I think Jim probably sensed that I needed help, but he was back at work trying to make up for all the time he had missed earlier that spring and summer. Plus, the neurologists kept telling him that there was nothing wrong with me. Jim's parents offered to pay for a live-in nanny to help with the boys, which might relieve some of my stress. Jim asked around and soon hired a woman who was probably in her early to midthirties. And for a few weeks she did, indeed, keep the boys and me alive, keep the house from burning down, and most likely she prevented several major catastrophes. However, she was a devout Christian, and when she came upon Jim's extensive stash of pornography, she told him she could no longer work in our home.

Suddenly Benjamin, Patrick, and I were on our own once again. I would wake up each morning with no memory of what had occurred the previous day. I recognized Jim and the boys simply because I saw them every day, but I would have no recollection of what any of us had done the day before, or what the plan was for that new day. Each day the world beyond my front door was an absolute unknown. Jim says that our family was full of *Lord of the Flies* incidents, in that he never knew exactly what he would come home to after work each day. Would I be there with Benjamin and Patrick? Would we all be gone? Would the boys be playing together in the backyard all by themselves with me nowhere in sight? Would I be there, but have no idea where Benjamin or Patrick were? Would the bath tub be overflowing? Would the oven or stove be on? Would the car be running in the driveway? I am terrified when I think about what that must have been like for the boys and me. I honestly do not know how we all survived those first days, weeks, months, and even years.

Part of the key to our survival may have been that my life quickly became governed by a very specific routine and a precise daily schedule. Most people find a certain amount of comfort in their day-to-day habits, and I suppose we all have a particular order that we like to do things in in our daily lives, whether it is a certain morning routine, or when, where, and with whom we like to eat our meals during the day, or our daily work schedules at the office. On the other hand, most people don't have a serious meltdown or mental collapse if they sleep through their alarm one morning, or if they have to push their lunchtime meeting to the following day. I would freak out about far less. If it was time for the boys and me to take our daily walk, and it was suddenly storming outside . . . I would be lost, and not know what I was supposed to do instead. If we lost power in the house during the time my schedule allotted for doing laundry, I would begin to sob. My daily routine was vital because it was all I knew. We had a gigantic wall calendar filled with pictures and stickers. The calendar carefully scripted out activities for the kids and me, and I would consult it to find out what we were supposed to be doing from one hour to the next. If a new task was introduced and I carefully worked it into my routine, I could repeat it and remember it. But God forbid I should ever reach the end of my to-do list before the end of the day. Without my list, I would be totally discombobulated. I wouldn't have any "next move." The opposite was true as well. If Jim came home from work and I had not yet completed everything that was planned for that day, I would again become totally distraught. Jim understands now that back in early years after the accident, the notion that I would actually have a say in what I could do simply didn't occur to me, and even if it did, the idea may have terrified me.

My mom wanted desperately to help out somehow, as well as give Jim a break. But my younger brother, Mark, was still living at home and was not yet driving. Mom felt like she couldn't very well desert him to come to Fort Worth to look after me. Instead it was decided that Jim would drive Benjamin, Patrick, and me to Houston to stay with my parents for a week. My parents now feel incredibly guilty about how little they understood of my new reality. My mom says that all she really knew was that I had this head injury and that I had trouble remembering things. The letters I sent her looked as if a first grader had written them, "all phonetic misspellings and shaky script on lined paper," but still she and my dad were not overly concerned.

It is highly unlikely that I in fact recognized either of my parents when I climbed out of the car in their driveway. But because Jim had prepared me for this particular reunion, I was able to greet them both with a sort of affection and warmth. Even so, both my parents say that they noticed immediately how much I had changed. They had known me as the family troublemaker, loud, defiant, and stubborn. Now my personality was completely different.

My dad was surprised at how cooperative and friendly I appeared, nothing like the person I had been even a few months earlier.

Mom thinks it likely that I woke up every morning that week in Houston unsure of where I was or why I was there. I must have been terribly confused to be yet again in a new, unfamiliar place, with unfamiliar people. But Mom thinks I would eventually hear the familiar sounds of Benjamin and Patrick, and then I would slowly find my bearings, and greet my parents as if nothing was amiss.

Not that everything went smoothly that week. Mom remembers taking me to a fancy luncheon and fashion show at a ritzy yacht club in the tony Houston suburb of Clear Lake. There were white linen tablecloths on the tables, and waiters in tuxedos. The only person I vaguely knew at this affair was my mother, but she recalls that I "did a good job of making conversation and acting normal." In the car afterward as we were driving home Mom claims I looked at her and said, "That's the dumbest thing I have ever done." Mom thinks I had no clue as to what had just happened. Or why. Why on earth had we gone to this place and eaten this meal? After all, it is entirely possible that I had never eaten anywhere except at a table in a house.

My dad remembers something else peculiar about that visit. I wouldn't even enter the backyard, because of the pool. I was absolutely petrified of that pool. He and my mom found that surprising, since I had always been a strong swimmer and loved the water. I had even been lifeguard as a teenager. Once again, they seemed not to understand the extent of my impairment. Nobody could comprehend that I was a different person, a new person, just observing and learning stuff as I went along. I seriously doubt I even understood my own fear of my parents' pool.

Because I was so deathly afraid of the pool out back, and wouldn't go near it, we usually spent the hottest part of the day with the boys in the second-floor family game room playing with toys that had belonged to us Miller kids years before. One afternoon I walked over to the piano and sat down. It was the same piano that I had learned to play on as a child. I placed my fingers on the keyboard and began playing Scott Joplin's "The Entertainer." Mom says I played it nearly flawlessly from start to finish. From memory.

When I was through, I turned to Mom and asked, "What was that? Where did that come from?" Mom told me that "The Entertainer" was a song that I had learned for a recital as a child. I was not able to ever repeat that performance. It was just gone. A kind of doorway had been opened momentarily, and then just as quickly, it was ruthlessly closed.

My brain was not in the habit of bestowing such gifts. Instead it was more often inclined to take away. During that same visit to Houston, Mom remembers coming upon me lying on the floor in the family room behind the wet bar. She thought it was an odd place for me to take a nap, but when she saw my eyes were open, she became alarmed. My parents weren't used to my lightning, but Benjamin, who was just two at the time, said something like, "Oh, it's all right, Grandma. She'll wake up in a few minutes." It happened again later in the week. My dad arrived home from work one evening, walked into the kitchen, and found me curled up in the corner of the large walk-in pantry. He looked at Mom and said, "What's going on?" Mom replied, "She did this earlier. Just leave her alone and in a little while she'll get up and come out of it."

All that week I kept asking for Jim several times a day. But

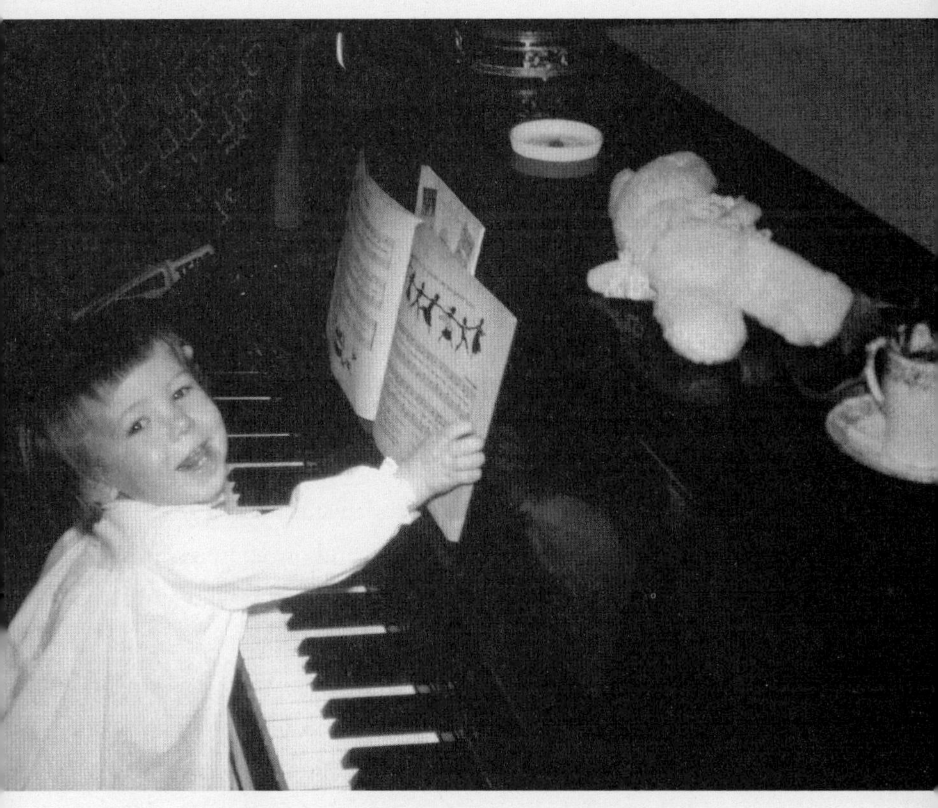

Me at my parents' piano. After my accident I would later play "The Entertainer" by heart on it.

when he finally did arrive the following Saturday afternoon, my mom says I had no idea who he was; in fact, I was afraid of him. Jim says he saw in my eyes instantly that I had once again forgotten him. Of course he was upset by that realization, but what could he do? Apparently, I made my younger brother, Mark, come with us on a walk that evening, because I did not want to be alone with this tall, curly-headed stranger.

~

A few days after returning home to Fort Worth, Jim sat down with me and taught me how to shave my legs. In fact, he taught me (and retaught me again and again and again) most of what I know about personal grooming. Come to think of it, Jim taught me pretty much everything I know about almost everything. Several weeks (or maybe it was months) later, there was even an awkward conversation about sex. I didn't exactly understand when he tried to explain what it meant to be a "mother" to Benjamin and Patrick. And being a "wife" to Jim was even more beyond my comprehension.

I suppose once upon a time, three years before, Jim and I had fallen in love. After the accident, I had no concept of "love." I knew Jim was there, and I quickly became dependent on him, and later became dependent on the boys, but I didn't really know him very well. I didn't know the most basic things about him, like what he enjoyed doing in his spare time, what his favorite foods were, what genre of books he liked to read, what music he liked to listen to, and hundreds of other little details. I can't be certain, but I don't think I even really cared so much about any of that stuff, either. I wasn't aware that I was supposed to care. However, Jim somehow still loved me. He still knew me, or at least the "me" I had been, which still looked like me. He knew everything about me; what I liked to do, eat, read, listen to, as well as every other trivial detail. But was I still that same Su? Hell no! Not by a long shot!

Jim loves telling me the following story:

> I knew something was terribly wrong between you and me, but I could never put my finger on it. And then one day it hit me. It was less than a year after the accident. We had just kissed, and I felt you pull away with a look in your eyes that I had seen before but had never comprehended. You no longer had a husband, a lover, or an equal partner in an adult relationship. You didn't get what any of those things meant. Instead, I was someone you could lean on. I was someone who could explain and teach things to you. Our relationship was no longer marital—instead it was familial. And the look on your face after that kiss was a look of discomfort, awkwardness, and even a little disgust. I was no longer your husband. I was more like a big brother. And it felt wrong somehow for you to kiss your big brother *that way*.

Jim remembered our love from before the accident, and he missed it. He tells me that when we were back at Ohio Wesleyan, we "went from friends to friends-with-benefits, to a committed and exclusive relationship." He talks about how he and I "would finish each other's sentences." He says we were inseparable and "when we were together, we were simply more." And now that particular Su that Jim had known was gone. I was utterly naive not only sexually, but emotionally as well. I just wasn't ready for such adult feelings, and wouldn't be for a few years.

5

You've Got A Friend

—James Taylor

Michele Hargett had been my college roommate at Ohio Wesleyan my sophomore year, and my maid of honor at my wedding. She is still one of my best friends. Michele wanted me to return the favor and come to South Carolina and be a bridesmaid at her wedding to Lynn Abbott in the fall of 1988. She knew of my injury and hospitalization. Jim tried to explain to her just how much I had lost, and how different I was. With the exception of driving from Fort Worth to my parents' house in Houston, I had never gone on any trips since my injury. I certainly had never been on an airplane. But it was decided that we would all drive to Jim's parents' house in Cedartown, Georgia, and then fly me up to Charleston, where the wedding was to be held. Jim would spend the week in Cedartown, and then drive up the following weekend for the ceremony, leaving the boys with his parents. Michele mentioned to me much later that she recalls asking Jim if I was going to be able to handle coming, and Jim reassuring her, "We're good."

Jim tried to prepare me for a plane flight from Atlanta to Charleston. He carefully explained the concept of a numbered seat, and where my luggage would go when the airline people took it. Who knows for sure what exactly happened on that flight. Maybe I blacked out and people just thought I was sleeping. Maybe I was totally obnoxious, asking my poor seat mate or the flight attendant a million questions. Maybe I cried because I didn't know what was happening or where I was going. Maybe I was totally silent, sitting there gripping the arms of my seat hoping for somebody familiar to show up and tell me what to do. Fortunately, Michele was waiting right there at the gate at the Charleston airport. Jim had warned her that I most likely would not know who she was, but surprisingly, I seemed to recognize her. Michele thinks that Jim must have prompted me with pictures, or maybe I just saw someone coming toward me with outstretched arms. Michele says, "We shared a big hug!"

She had been playing tennis one day in May of 1988 when a mutual friend told her about my injury. "She had the funniest accident. A ceiling fan fell on her head." Michele recalls feeling sick. "I think I sent a care package she recalls." But she didn't realize the extent of the damage until she received my first letter. "It was a thank-you letter, thanking me for the package I had sent," she remembers. "What shocked me wasn't the content of the letter, it was how basic it was. The level was just so low, and you were just always so brilliant, so intelligent. And that was the first time it jarred me as to how serious this was."

At her parents' house in Charleston, Michele and I slept together in a queen-size bed in one of the guest bedrooms.

"I'd get up and start moving around each morning," Michele recalls. "And every single day, the whole week before the wedding, the first words out of your mouth were, 'Where's Jim?' And I would say, 'Jim's back home with the kids.' And then I'd ask, 'Do you know who I am? And you'd say, 'No.' And then I'd say, 'I'm Michele Hargett. I'm your college roommate from Ohio Wesleyan, and you are here for my wedding.' And then, as you got up and going, it was like everything settled back into place, and you would lose your 'glazed' look. You would eventually know where you were, and why you were there, but only the most basic stuff."

Michele made lists of things that had changed about me since the accident: Red was still my favorite color. I had the same quirky sense of humor. I still had "that likability factor." But all of the history of our friendship was gone. "All the funny things that before would have had you on the floor laughing . . . now it was just a blank stare. You know how when the power goes out, you walk into a room and still turn on the light switch, and each time you're surprised when it doesn't come on? That's what it was like. Each time, it was like a slap in the face. Oh, yeah, she doesn't remember that." Other things that Michele noticed: I had smoked sporadically, at parties mostly, in college. Now I thought it was the most disgusting habit. Before I had a horribly rocky relationship with my parents, and now I spoke of them with the greatest love and respect.

Michele noticed that when Jim arrived, I seemed "whole" again. She says, "It was almost as if the accident had never happened." On Michele's wedding day, she and I put on Rollerblades and Jim towed us behind his car.

I have no memories of that week, or of Michele and Lynn's wedding.

~

When Christmas came that year, Jim, Benjamin, Patrick, and I drove to Houston. During my childhood, Christmas in the Miller household had been full of rituals and traditions. Now I seemed to be lost and totally baffled by nearly everything that was said and done. My mom told me, "It was obvious from your manner that you were confused by this whole holiday season." I was confused by why so many members of the family who weren't usually together were all together now. I didn't understand why we were going to church at night, and why we were eating all of these special meals. And I was very confused as to why there were so many different kinds of cookies, why there was not one, but two trees inside my parents' house, and why there were so many decorations everywhere. Jim must have done all our Christmas shopping and wrapping that year.

Mom thinks that my sister Diane and her husband, Paul, were there that year, because their daughter, Kaitlin, had been born the same September as Patrick, in 1987, so the two baby cousins, along with Benjamin, were all going to have Christmas at Grandma's. I had not "met" Diane yet, since the injury. I'm told that every time I walked into a room where she was, I would walk up to her and say, "You must be Diane. You're one of my sisters."

The whole Miller family, whenever they get together, always laugh about and share the same stories about "growing up Miller." Stories about neighbors and neighborhoods, stories about teachers we all had in school, stories about unfairly getting in trouble, and who was really responsible for breaking that window. The anecdotes are never-ending, and I'm sure this Christmas was no exception. All of this bonding, all of the inside jokes and stories, used to drive me absolutely crazy! I didn't feel as if I was a part of this family at all. I didn't understand the stories and so couldn't contribute to them. And when everyone laughed and joked, I felt like they were all laughing at me, even though I know now that they weren't.

Over the years both my parents began to notice that when the family was gathered for some big occasion and the conversation turned to the past, I would either get up and leave the room, or simply try to change the subject. For years I had no comprehension about what all I didn't know. And until very recently, I wasn't at all interested in looking at slides or photo albums. I wonder now if all of those old pictures were some kind of reminder to me about how much I was missing and in some way what a huge empty space there was in my life.

Very gradually, my ability to form new memories seemed to improve. Barb and her husband, Scott, visited us in Texas the following spring, a year after the accident. Barb remembers that I still was having a lot of really bad headaches. "You were swigging Diet Cokes constantly to try to keep the headaches away." But she also noticed some positive changes. She said that I recognized her, and I seemed to know where I was. She remembers thinking that my tastes in both music and food had changed. I was always a picky eater, and Barb was surprised by some of the foods I was eating. But I question now, Had my tastes really changed, or had I simply figured out after just a year how to get along and act the way people expected me to?

There are always more questions than there are answers.

6

Eminence Front

—The Who

During the spring of 1989, I still wasn't doing too well. I may have started making new memories, or at least appearing to, but nothing that doctors had told Jim about me regaining my past memories was happening. Nothing was coming back. This made any social situations extremely awkward, especially with people who had known me before. Jim says we began to avoid doing anything with any other people because it was just too hard on everyone involved. Many of our friends told Jim it was as if I had died, and some kind of weird impostor, who looked exactly like me, had taken my place. At church, at the fitness center, and even in the neighborhood, the way that I now interacted with people made them feel nervous and uncomfortable. I didn't always notice, but if I did, I didn't understand why they felt that way. I also didn't get why people apparently pitied Jim, the boys, and me. I didn't like to be touched and hugged by people who I wasn't at all familiar with, which, sadly, was nearly everyone as far as I was concerned. With the exception of Jim, Benjamin, Patrick, my parents, my younger brother, and possibly one or two others, everyone was a stranger.

But really, I was the stranger. I didn't know when I was acting peculiar. I didn't realize that I constantly repeated myself, and often acted just like a child. It took me a long time to process information, so I had a hard time answering questions and keeping up with the normal rhythm of an ordinary conversation. It was also confusing and frightening when people would shout at me. If it took me too long to answer a question, for example, people would often repeat themselves using a much louder voice, as if they thought my hearing was somehow impaired. Jim was heartbroken to see me struggling so much. And he felt bad for our friends, who were just trying to understand and help out any way they could. I was obviously frustrated, often scared, and even sometimes rude to people. And there was still a certain vacant look in my eyes that never seemed to go away.

The previous January, Jim had taken the advice of one of my neurologists, who suggested I try going back to college at Texas Christian University. The doctor thought that the structure of school, as well as the classes themselves, might force my brain to "wake up." Jim, willing to try anything, enrolled me in a few 100-level classes. He believes he may have even spoken to the professors, explaining the situation as best he could: trying to go to school was going to be a challenge for me. In the mornings before leaving for work, Jim would drive the boys to their Montessori preschool, and then drop me off at the campus.

I seriously have to question the rationale behind this little experiment. What exactly were these people thinking sending me off to be a college student? I couldn't even read. I could barely write. I was totally socially unaware and inept. What did I even do when I was in class? Did I understand what was going on? How did I act around other college-age students and professors? And how stupid was it that we paid full tuition for this craziness? Maybe it's a good thing that I don't remember! But even though I don't remember it, I am angry when I hear that I was put through something like this. And that a *doctor* suggested such a thing. This charade came to a grinding halt some weeks later. Jim remembers that someone found me sitting on a bench on campus, sobbing. I didn't know where I was. That person was somehow able to get in contact with Jim at work. He came and picked me up and took me home. That was the end of my education at TCU.

In May, Jim planned another, more appropriate "experiment" by way of a family trip to Sea World in San Antonio, Texas. He desperately wanted things—meaning me—to get back to normal. He thought a low-key, typical suburban family vacation would help. Jim knew that I had gone to Sea World with my family when I was younger, and he thought that putting me in what might be a familiar environment could possibly spark some Su-type memories. At least that is what he hoped for. In one photograph from that trip, Benjamin and Patrick are sitting in strollers shaped like whales. They are wearing matching outfits and have matching haircuts. They could almost be twins. Pictures such as these are often all I have, because I certainly don't remember that vacation.

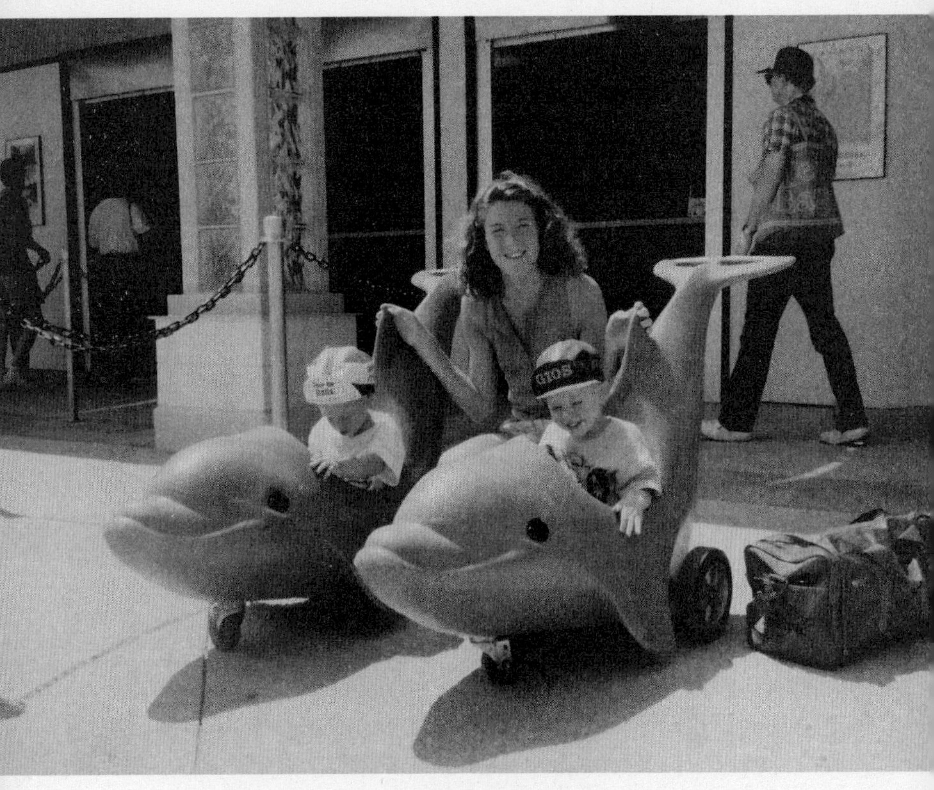

Patrick, Benjamin, and me at SeaWorld—a Nice Normal Family Vacation, San Antonio, Texas, 1989

I can, however, repeat the stories of that trip after having been told them again and again. Apparently, at one point Jim lifted Patrick up so he could see the dolphins better, and so he could pet them. Patrick immediately started screaming and struggling to get out of Jim's arms, so Jim set him down. When Jim asked him what was wrong, it turned out that Benjamin had told Patrick, "You better watch out because Mommy and Dad are going to feed you to those big fish." Benjamin's precocious intellect, developed as a result of my dependency on him, was unfortunately the bane of Patrick's young existence. This incident was reminiscent of another, one earlier that spring while they were playing together in the sandbox in the backyard. Benjamin told his little brother that fire ants tasted like purple Skittles. Poor Patrick ended up with a horrendously sore and swollen mouth and tongue.

It was after that excursion to Sea World that Jim began to seriously consider moving away from Texas. I failed to remember ever having been at such a memorable place, and I think he was a little bit disappointed about that. Jim thought a fresh start somewhere else might be good for everyone in the family.

Jim had been with General Dynamics for almost four years. He was only twenty-five, but he already possessed highly marketable skills in the aerospace and defense industry. He told me that his market value as an engineer would be higher somewhere else. He said he was considering looking for a job on the East Coast; perhaps New England or somewhere in the mid-Atlantic, like Baltimore or Washington, D.C. I'm sure that I hadn't a clue as to what he was talking to me about, but it was decided that he would interview with a few places and then we would move. He ended up accepting a job at Allied Signal in Baltimore, Maryland. Jim says

Patrick's second birthday in September. The next problem was somehow figuring out a way to get two cars, two kids, and two cats to Baltimore. Jim came up with what he thought was the most obvious solution: I would drive one car with the kids, and Jim would drive the other car with the cats. Jim outfitted both cars with CB radios, and showed me how to work mine so we could keep in contact with each other along the way. I agreed readily to his plan, just like I agreed with most everything he said back then. Jim thoroughly regrets the decision now. At the time, he thought there was no other option, but he also admits now that he didn't fully realize the extent of my confusion about almost everything. He told me recently that in the world of really dumb ideas he has had in his life, this was probably one of his worst.

Again, my actual memories of this mighty trip east are not at all clear, and I don't think Jim's recollections are much better. The journey was, however, not without incident. We were supposed to drive that first day all the way from Fort Worth to Jim's parents' house outside of Atlanta, and spend the night with them. But for whatever reason—maybe we got a late start—we ended up having to stop in rural Mississippi for the night. There was a bass-fishing tournament in whatever little off-the-highway town it was, and hotel rooms were extremely scarce. We ended up pulling into what looked to be a minimally acceptable motel (the rent-by-the-hour sort). Jim went into the office to ask someone about room availability while I waited with the boys, who were both asleep in their car seats by this point. Apparently, a very drunk bass fisherman opened the passenger-side door and crawled into my car. I have no idea what he said to me. I can sort of recall the smell of him and being frozen in place, not able to talk or move, but nothing else. Jim came back from the office and found me shaking like a leaf, nearly in tears. I was barely able to speak and explain to him what had happened. He was chilled to the bone when he realized what I was trying to say: *There was a man. He was drunk. He smelled bad. He said something. I was scared. Then he went away.* I sometimes wonder what really took place in my car. Certainly Jim would not have been gone long enough for anything too terrible to happen. Right? We ended up staying for what was left of the night in a tiny, moldy, foul-smelling room. I'm curious as to whether I slept at all.

The next morning we got back on the road and made it to Jim's parents' house by late afternoon. After a much more comfortable nights' sleep at their place, we pressed on to what we thought would be our final leg to Baltimore. But we hadn't driven too far when Jim's car broke down outside of Charlotte in Concord, N.C. This car was one that he had purchased from my parents, and it had been driven for years by several of the Miller children, myself included. Jim says that there was a crack in the transmission housing, and he fed it transmission fluid regularly. But the car had chosen this particular morning, to seize up. Jim left the boys and me at a Burger King and headed to a nearby service station. Benjamin and Patrick were initially thrilled to be out of their car seats, and they entertained themselves in that Burger King playland for quite some time, jumping and running around while I sat and watched. One hour stretched to two, then to four, then to six. They both got hot, tired, hungry, and cranky. And I imagine I was pretty tired and cranky myself. I didn't have any money to buy them food and drinks. Jim had told me to "Stay here!" in that certain tone of voice he had. And because I was a little bit afraid of him when he used that certain tone of voice, I did what I was told.

It turned out the car could not be fixed. Jim called his new boss in Baltimore, who suggested that Jim rent a truck and tow the car. The only rental available in town when Jim inquired was a twenty-six-foot U-Haul. He came and told me all of this at the Burger King, where I had been sitting with a two- and three-year-old for almost eight hours. Jim remembers me telling him that I didn't care what we did next but that whatever it was, the kids were going to be his! I wanted nothing more to do with either of them for a *very* long time!

It was nearly evening at this point, and none of us really wanted to drive anywhere except to a hotel for the night. Unfortunately, there was a huge NASCAR event going on at the Charlotte Motor Speedway, so there were no hotel rooms to be found. We kept going, on to the next town, and the next, but everything for miles around was booked. It soon got dark, and the oncoming headlights on Interstate 85 began to bewilder me. This kind of sensory overload, along with being thoroughly exhausted, was precisely the worst scenario for me, the exact kind of situation that would cause me to shut down. We were approaching a busy interchange at Interstate 40. I became confused and chose the wrong lane, heading west toward Tennessee. Jim, trying to navigate the road with the enormous U-Haul that was towing our dead car, didn't immediately notice that I was no longer behind him. He had gone several miles before he glanced in the rearview mirror and saw, to his horror, that I wasn't there. He reached for his CB radio and turned up the volume. Immediately he heard a group of truckers declaring, "This crazy lady on the radio has hijacked channel ten and keeps asking for 'Jim'!" Jim picked up the receiver and called out for me. I recognized his voice and he asked me what I could see, so he could try to figure out where I was. Unfortunately, I was panicking, and for a while I didn't make much sense. I have no idea how, but Jim says that eventually he was able to calm me

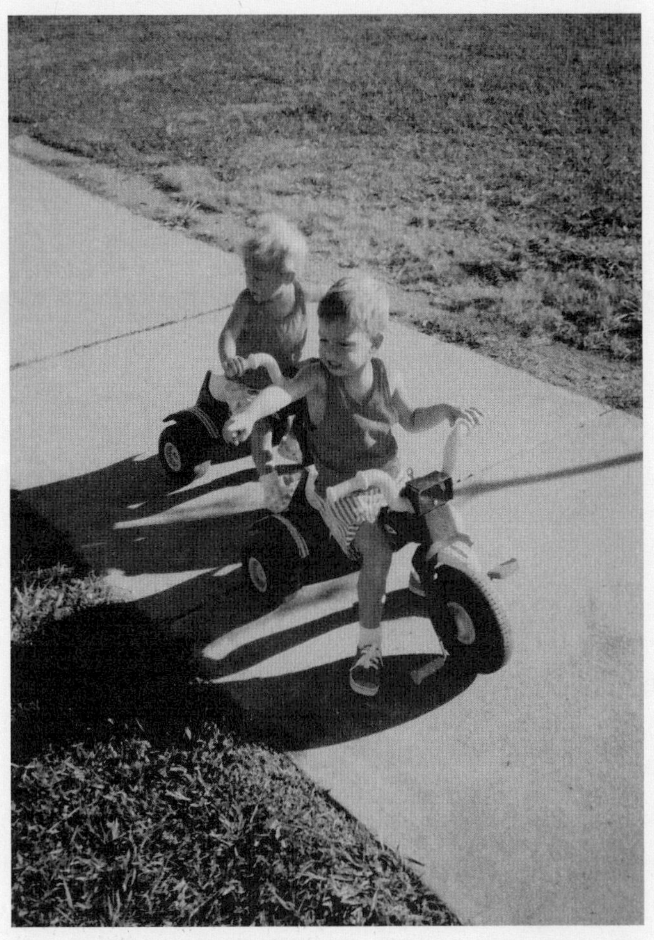

Benjamin and Patrick on their blue tricycles. Having seen this photo may be part of why I remember those days more clearly than others.

down, and ultimately talk me through exiting I-40 and making my way back to I-85. I still think it is a not so small miracle that I was able to follow his directions and, in the end, locate him. How was it that I was able to keep it together enough to even drive, let alone follow his directions? It makes no sense. Like so many things in my life, how did I ever live to tell the tale?

The following day we rolled into the parking lot of the Welcome Inn in Towson, Maryland, our home for the next several weeks until we could close on the house we had bought in Bel Air. Jim remembers arriving late at night, exhausted after days of driving. I have only the vaguest of memories of the whole time we lived there: carrying laundry down to the Laundromat that was at the bottom of a long hill, and the boys flying down that hill on their blue Fisher-Price tricycles, watching all the different-colored Disney "Sing-Along Songs" videos, and looking at books with the boys. I have no idea what Benjamin, Patrick, and I did to fill those days. Did I know where I was? Did the boys and I ever try to venture out anywhere? If so, how did we find our way back? Did I rely on Benjamin? Did I understand that I was no longer in Texas? Basically, everything I knew was gone again, and Jim thinks that the boys and I just sat in our room every day waiting for him to come back. He doesn't remember me complaining about the situation, or showing any outward signs of stress, so he didn't worry too much until one evening when he came home and found me in a state that he hadn't seen before. He says that I had "lost it, like catatonia, lost it!" He says that I was awake but "checked out, unresponsive, just withdrawn, like PTSD." I spoke, but only if I was spoken to first. He says I looked "stunned, or in shock."

Had something terrible happened that day? I don't know. These are the kinds of stories that freak me out a little bit more each time I hear them. Again, how the hell did I survive? How did my kids survive in my care? What kinds of things did Benjamin and Patrick see me do? What did they think of me? Or was my erratic, inconsistent, and childlike behavior normal to them? Was this just the way Mommy was?

Jim called his new boss, Bill, and explained the situation. Bill said that Jim should contact the Employee Assistance Program, which he did. After that phone call, Jim decided to take me to a psychiatric hospital. He thinks that all this happened on a Friday, and that I may have spent the weekend there while they did a psychiatric evaluation. The results came back showing that I was not suicidal, and not a threat to the kids. I was more lucid by Sunday, asking Jim, "Why am I here?" He thinks, looking back, that everything just got to be too much for me. I must have been so confused about what was going on since leaving Texas. Too much change, too quickly, and Jim not knowing how badly off I really was. Unfortunately, this was not the last time that I would be uprooted and set down in a new and confusing place.

8

Mama, I'm Comin' Home

—Ozzy Osbourne

We moved out of the Welcome Inn and into our house right around Halloween in 1989. The house was a small two-story colonial with three bedrooms, a finished basement, and a one-car garage at the end of a cul-de-sac called Kingsmark Court. By the end of that day Benjamin had dumped the tricycle and was instead riding his red two-wheeler around and around the circle right in front of our new house at top speed, with Patrick trying to keep up on his trike. Obviously the weeks we spent cooped up in a motel room had not had any negative effects on them whatsoever. I, however, struggled with learning a new house. Jim remembers me having to keep all the cupboards and drawers opened in the kitchen for several weeks—possibly months—before relearning where things were kept. It drove him crazy, and he often shouted at me because it meant the boys had open access to everything from knives and scissors to pots and pans, canned food, and opened boxes of cereal. Another issue: my washing machine and dryer in Texas had been right off the kitchen, and in this house they were in the basement. I would forget that I even had a basement, so I would think there were no washer and dryer. Then I would get upset with Jim and complain, "Jim, why did we buy this house? There isn't even a washing machine or dryer!"

The house in Bel Air is the first house that we lived in that I sort of remember, but even here, the memories I have are more impressions. We bought the boys new bunk beds from Cargo Furniture. Benjamin slept on the top bunk, Patrick on the bottom, although there were some mornings when they would be curled up together on the top bunk. As soon as Patrick turned two, he wanted to do everything Benjamin did. They were inseparable for many years.

We started attending Bel Air United Methodist Church on Sunday mornings, and Jim and I both sang in the choir. On Wednesday evenings we went to choir practice, and a few of those fellow choristers became our friends. Socializing, for me still remained puzzling. Jim talks about me being confused whenever we were invited to somebody's house for dinner. I usually asked him at some point during the drive home, "What was that all about?" A woman named Janet White, was probably the youngest member of the adult choir at the church, along with Jim and me, so we sort of gravitated toward each other and became good friends. Janet was single and a math teacher at the local high school. She would come over to our house for meals and movie nights. One time I made blueberry pancakes. But instead of buying what I thought were blueberries at the grocery store, I had gotten little grapes. With seeds. It was a difficult, messy ordeal trying to eat pancakes with seeds. She says she still laughs when she thinks about it. She and Jim both loved the Monty Python movies, and had most of them practically memorized. At the time, I never quite understood the humor, so I couldn't really share in the experience with them. Nonetheless, Janet had an easygoing personality and more than tolerated Benjamin and Patrick, so I felt comfortable with her.

It was about a year after first meeting her that Jim and I told her about my accident. When I asked her recently about what she thought when we first told her the story, she remarked, "I was amazed, because you and Jim seemed like this perfect couple with these lovely children. I specifically remember Jim describing how you didn't remember him, and you didn't remember the boys. And I remember you talking about your bewilderment initially as to who all these people were. I was amazed at how much you appeared totally normal. It wasn't until it was just you and I, or the two of us with Jim, that you would kind of reveal things you didn't understand. You weren't really opening up to anyone. It was like, 'I don't want to look like an idiot.' "

Because there were rarely other adults around to help me, Jim sat down with Benjamin at some point and taught him how to tell time and how to read a map even before he could read books. "It started out as a game that Dad and I played. Dad would give me a location, the name of a place, like the grocery store and I would have to find out how to get there. It progressed to streets and even intersections that I had to find. I was always the navigator for many years." Benjamin recalls. "Whether I was in the front seat or the backseat of the car, I would have the map on my lap. If we had to go somewhere new, it was my job to find it on the map, and then

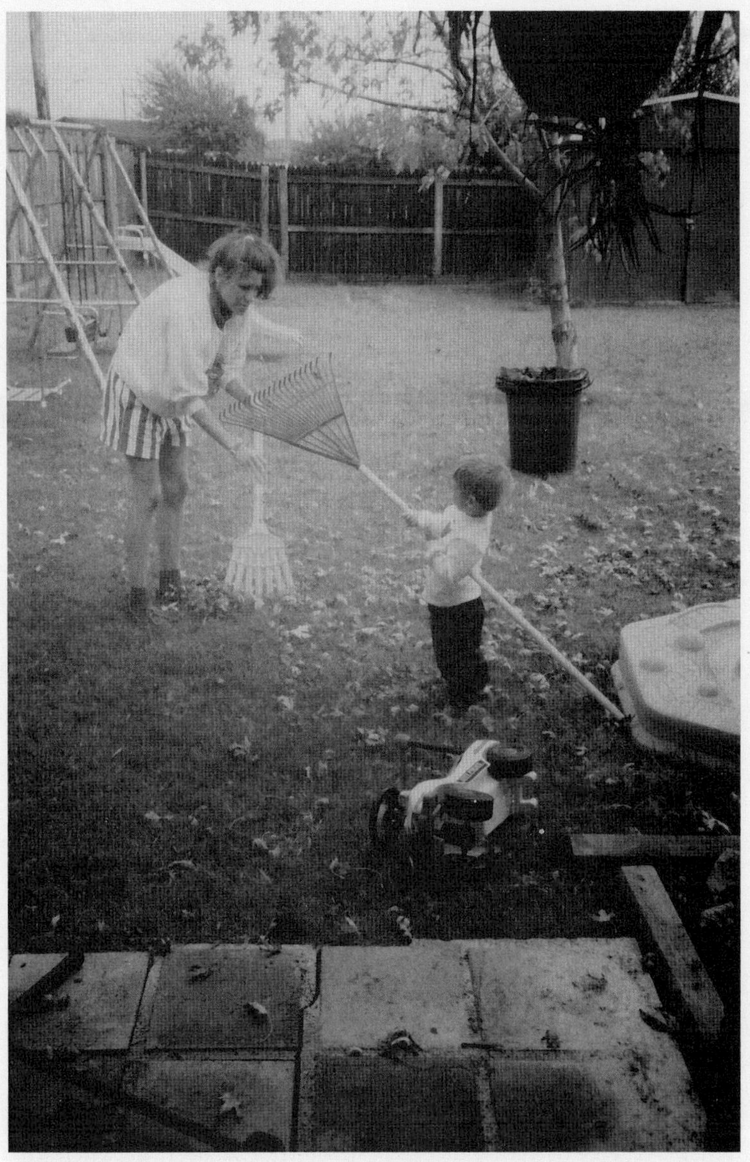

Benjamin and I raking leaves in our back yard in Fort, Worth, Texas.
Notice who has the big rake and who has the child-size rake.

tell you where to go. It never felt like a responsibility. It was more exciting than that. Nothing about it seemed like a job or a chore. More like a mission." He was three.

I slowly began to learn my way around, but continued to depend on three-year-old Benjamin to help me navigate when Jim wasn't around. I was terrified to drive on the highway after the long frightening drive up from Texas, so Benjamin learned the back roads to get us from one place to another. I think that both Jim and I started about this time to look to Benjamin as "head of the household" when Jim was away. Benjamin definitely had very different skills from most other three-year-olds. He was very verbal, with an enormous vocabulary, but he was also very physically coordinated. He learned to ride his two-wheeler just after turning three, and he was fearless when it came to almost everything! It wasn't until he was much older that Benjamin realized he had done many unusual things for his age as a little kid. He talks about how he remembers sitting down with me at the kitchen table and helping with the grocery lists. At the grocery store, he remembers helping put Patrick in the seat in the cart, and then holding my hand as we navigated our way together up and down the aisles. He says, "It didn't seem weird, because it was the way things had always been."

Every morning Benjamin would ask me something like, "What's going to happen today?" or "What's our plan?" And we would go through the day together. "Maybe we could go to the library today. Or maybe you can take a walk. You can push Patrick in the stroller while I ride my bike." He was helpful with Patrick, remembering where his juice was in the refrigerator, or where his diapers were located. He was horrible about picking up his toys, or getting ready for bed at night, but he had some pretty intense survival skills, and he wasn't afraid of anything. Jim says now that he was worried back then about me having one of my "lightning strikes" in the car while driving with the boys. And apparently I did, although Benjamin is the only one who remembers these incidents. He says, "There were a few times when we would be going somewhere and you would pull over, and we'd have to sit for a while." I would say to the boys, "I'm going to lie down for a minute." And I would lie down with my hands over my head. Did I not tell Jim about these episodes on purpose, or did I honestly forget they had happened by the time he got home? Benjamin and Patrick somehow knew that they shouldn't tell him when stuff like that happened, either. I was afraid of doing almost everything back then. But I was more afraid of Jim.

9

The Great Pretender

—Queen

Jim doesn't remember us ever sitting down and having a specific conversation about how we weren't going to tell people about my injury and the implications it continued to have for my life. Instead, it was just understood that there would be no discussions about it with any of our new neighbors and friends. We did tell a few very close friends, over the years, a sort of shortened, watered-down version, making the whole experience seem far less serious and far more humorous than it was and continued to be. I don't honestly know why, exactly. Was I embarrassed? Was Jim embarrassed? Did Jim really think that there was nothing wrong with me anymore, and that I was totally back to normal? Did he *have* to think that way in order to be able to leave the boys with me each day? I am sure we both wanted more than anything for everything to just be normal.

In September 1990, we enrolled Benjamin in a preschool program at our Methodist church. The following month, his teacher asked if I wanted to help chaperone the trip to the pumpkin patch and farm. I declined. I just couldn't do it. Chaperoning a fieldtrip was something I had never done before, and I might have been afraid of doing it wrong. I was constantly afraid of doing things wrong. But unfortunately, I did stuff wrong all the time. And Jim didn't let me forget it. If I tried to change the bag on the vacuum cleaner, and ended up with dirt everywhere because I had installed it incorrectly; if I forgot to get bread, or eggs, or chips, or whatever Jim specifically asked me to get at the store; if Jim got a call at work from Benjamin's preschool teacher that I forgot to pick Benjamin up that day; if I got lost coming home from the library, and at 6:30 I still hadn't started dinner; if I mistakenly used bathroom cleaner instead of furniture polish, on the wooden kitchen chairs and ruined a number of them; if I forgot to go to the dry cleaners to pick up Jim's shirts: If any things happened, it meant I was stupid.

I have tried countless times to put myself in Jim's shoes. It must have been more than a little infuriating to live with me. Our home should have been the place where he could relax, spend time with his kids, and carry on adult conversations with me. Our home was none of those things.

Our constant quest for normalcy made every event a high-stakes performance. As a way to illustrate this fact, I'll relate a story that we laugh about now, but at the time it was not at all amusing. That first Christmas we lived in Maryland, Jim thought it would be fun to go and chop down a tree to decorate for our new house. He had fond childhood memories of finding and cutting down the perfect Christmas tree with his family every December, and he wanted to start a new tradition with Patrick and Benjamin. So, off we went. Jim was carrying an ax and a saw. I was carrying Patrick and holding on to Benjamin's hand as we trudged through the snow. My boys and I had never seen snow before. When it snowed for the first time early that December, I can remember Benjamin, in his pajamas, barreling out onto the deck, full speed ahead, so loud and excited. While Patrick, more cautious, sat in the doorway for a bit, hunched down touching the flakes tentatively with his fingers, before walking out onto the deck cautiously. I can remember being a little confused as to why snow was both white and wet. I had seen pictures of snow, so I should have known it was white, but I didn't expect it to be *so* white and I don't know why, but I thought it would have a different consistency.

As we walked for what seemed like miles, I remember it being very cold and windy, and both boys' noses were running. Jim was all about finding the Ultimate Meck Family Christmas Tree. I was all about getting this over with so we could go home where it was warm. Jim was convinced that if we just kept looking, and walking just a little bit farther, we would find "our" tree. We eventually found what Jim was looking for, and he cut it down. Benjamin, of course, wanted to help with the ax and the saw and he ended up getting screamed at by Jim instead. Patrick was tired, cold, and whiny. The whole thing was quite the miserable adventure. Both boys fell asleep in their car seats while Jim was trying to tie the tree to the car, and we ended up not eating any of the special cutting-the-tree-down snacks we had prepared. Apparently, Jim remembered always having snacks *after* the tree was hunted and slain, and not *before*. He was upset that the boys and I hadn't appreciated this outing. I was upset because I hadn't seen the point of this outing.

I still needed routine desperately and I missed the aerobics classes that I had taken in Texas. So Jim and I joined Merritt Athletic Club, a fitness facility not too far from Jim's office. I made almost daily trips to that club and was noticed by Brenda Miller, the aerobics coordinator. She ultimately offered me a job teaching classes to the "Mom set" most mornings. I recently found an old VHS tape of me teaching one of those classes, wearing black Lycra shorts with a wide belt, a white jog bra, and thick white socks with high-top aerobics sneakers. My hair, which I seem to use as a prop, is long and curly, thanks to an early-nineties-era spiral perm.

I don't remember too much about teaching at Merritt. But I do recall a distinct feeling of satisfaction that I had being an aerobics instructor. Finally, I could help out financially, at least a little bit, and also feel like there was more to my life than being a wife and mother. Brenda Miller also started a dance team, Muscles in Motion, and I was thrilled when she asked me to be part of it.

It was while living in Bel Air, and teaching at Merritt, that I think I actively began to watch and listen to what other people did and said. Before this time, what I did was utterly instinctive. Now, after observing, I began, to mimic (exactly) how different people in different situations acted. Most, if not all of the time I didn't understand why people behaved certain ways in different circumstances, but that didn't matter to me. My number one goal was to fit in. I never wanted to say or do anything stupid. I rarely did anything because I thought it was the right thing to do; I just acted, literally, like those around me, whether at church, at the gym, at social gatherings, at the library, the playground, or with other neighbors. I mimicked movements, activities, gestures, speech patterns, and facial expressions. If all the mothers at the park were sitting with their legs crossed and flipping through magazines, I would cross my legs and flip through a magazine. If people in church were standing and singing a hymn, I would stand with my hymnal opened and pretend to sing the same hymn. It took me years to learn how to read, so I could barely follow along with the bulletin or the hymnal during services. In choir, I listened intently and paid attention during the rehearsals to the words and tunes of our music. I would then try to either follow along or memorize as much as I could. It was quite a few years before I realized the word *alleluia* wasn't *alligator,* and *amen* wasn't *a man,* and *let us pray* wasn't *lettuce rain.*

I also had dozens of my own made-up words and phrases that I used. My brother Rob recently reminded me of two of these that he explicitly remembers: "Long-end days" were what I called the weekend, as in: When *the long-end days* get here, we are going to go and visit Mom and Dad. And "real art" was how I referred to photographs, as in: I am going to pick up the *real art* from Moto Photo this afternoon.

Over the years, I have taken "blending in" to an Olympic-class level. This need I have to conform has taken its toll on me and has led to quite the exhausting existence. In Texas, Jim says that our friends had treated me as if I was suddenly mentally retarded. When we moved east I was treated, at least I thought, as if I belonged. Except I didn't, and I was the only one who knew the truth. As hard as I worked to fit in, one would think that I would be happy that I seemed to be succeeding. But the pressure was *always* on, and I was extremely self-conscious. I could never really relax and be *me* because I didn't know who that was. Who exactly was I supposed to be? It was almost like the "What Would Jesus Do?" expression that was popular a few years ago, except I was constantly asking myself "What Would Su Do?" Because I honestly didn't know how to think for myself. I just knew how to parrot others. I had no understanding or appreciation of why people did what they did. Or was *everybody* going through motions just like I was? I didn't think so.

For example, I was expected to attend the occasional social gathering with people from Jim's office. I hated going to those senseless functions. They were full of all these power people, with all of their college degrees, and PhDs, with important jobs and important lives. All the women knew how to dress perfectly and how do their hair and makeup just so. Nobody ever taught me how to do stuff like that. I felt totally intimidated! I sensed I was like a four- or five-year-old surrounded by grown-ups. I didn't fit in at all with these people no matter how hard I tried to imitate them. Often I would throw up while getting ready because I was so nervous and uncomfortable about going. And then Jim would get so pissed off at me.

He says now that he had no idea what I was going through. He never understood my reluctance. So our social life just became another source of anxiety and tension between the two of us. All Jim wanted was a bit of what we had before, "to go out and do things like we used to do." Except I didn't know what we used to do, and I was terrified of these social situations. I was also scared of being separated from Jim at these parties. I never knew what to say. The whole chitchatthing was beyond me. Women would gather in the kitchen and talk about their high-pressure jobs, their exotic vacations, what a pain in the ass it was to find a good au pair for their kids that they hated. I never had anything to contribute, so

I awkwardly stood around watching the clock and wishing time would go faster so Jim would come and find me and we could just go home. But as afraid as I was to go to these get-togethers, I was more frightened of provoking Jim's anger if I stood my ground and refused to go. There were times when he wouldn't forgive or talk to me for weeks if I did that. Jim wanted to act as if everything was back to normal. As part of the pact that we had seemingly made with each other to not talk about my injury with friends, neighbors, and Jim's coworkers, we also stopped talking to each other.

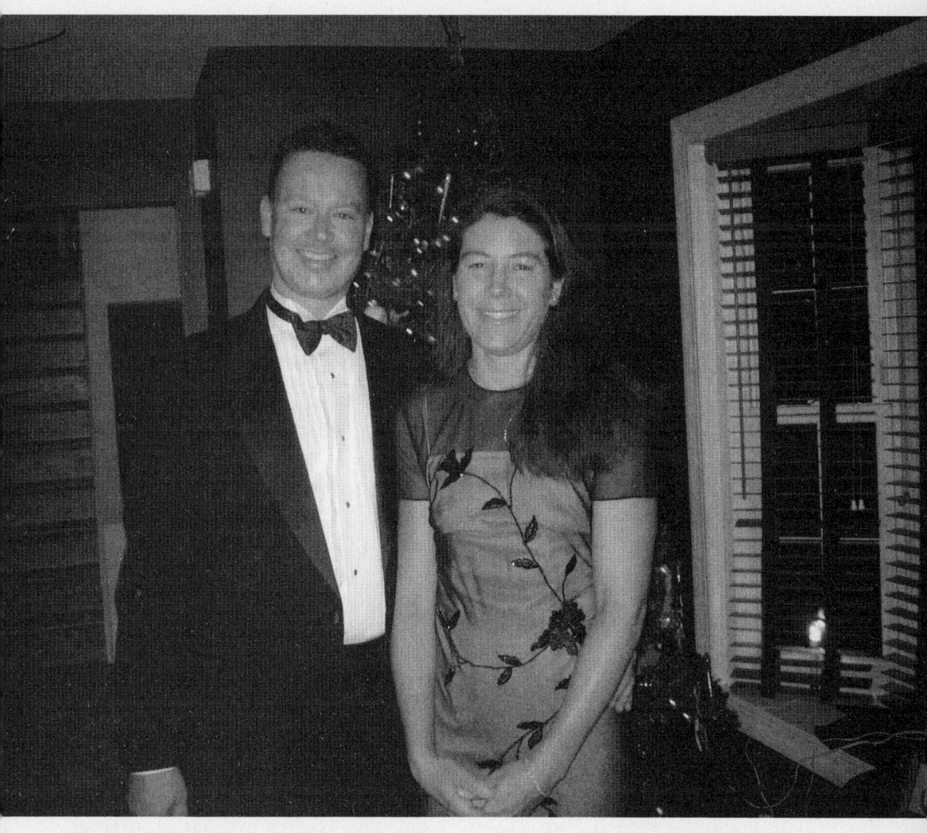

Headed out to a company Christmas party. I threw up right before this picture was taken, but then I had to put on my happy party face.

10

Life Is a Lemon, and I Want My Money Back

—Meatloaf

We had been living in Bel Air for almost a year when Benjamin started going to preschool. What I remember most about his preschool classroom was the strawberry wallpaper. Benjamin says he vividly remembers that wallpaper, too. Once, when the teachers weren't looking, he went over to the wallpaper, utterly convinced that when he scratched it, it would smell like strawberries, because of a scratch-and-sniff book we had read. Did I have the same urge? Who knows? I was more peer than parent to Patrick and Benjamin, both mentally and emotionally. I was filled with the same awe and wonder that they were about many aspects of the world.

Unfortunately, Benjamin's strong, take-no-prisoners personality, became a disadvantage as he started preschool, and it continued to be a liability throughout his school years. Early on he was put on a kind of preschool probation. There were these little yellow tags he would get at the end of each day labeled with the numbers one through five. Whatever number was circled represented how he had behaved that day. I think there was also a kind of an incentive system built into the yellow tags. So if he got a certain number of "fives" during the week, he was allowed to pick a sticker to take home on Friday. I remember thinking it was strange, and I was unsure as to what my role was with regard to these little yellow tags. I didn't know that I was supposed to talk to him about his behavior or discipline him somehow. I honestly don't think that Benjamin was a bad kid. The whole concept that he was somehow inferior to the teacher, I am convinced, was a bit baffling to him. When he was at home with Patrick and me there was an awful lot expected of him, but with all of those expectations came a certain amount of freedom. I depended on Benjamin to a certain extent to know what to do and when to do it. At school, that responsibility was mysteriously taken away from him, and the teacher, instead, got to pick what to do and when to do it. Most days Benjamin must have thought the four-year-old version of "Screw it! I feel like going outside on the playground now, and I could care less about sitting here quietly listening to you talk about the days of the week!"

Moreover, I didn't know too much about discipline, reverse psychology, or time-outs because I didn't remember being parented myself. Every day was a brand-new day to the boys and me. If there was a "rule" at home one day that stipulated "all books back on the bookshelf after bedtime reading," that rule would be totally forgotten by the next evening, when all three of us would fall asleep in the top bunk with a dozen or more books scattered about. If the boys got in serious trouble one day for walking into the house from the backyard with muddy boots on, the next time they wore their muddy boots in the house, I might not even notice. Benjamin says of that time: "Patrick and I were able to do pretty much what we wanted. Almost all of our free time when we were little was spent together. We played outside a lot and did all kinds of dangerous stuff. We would get into the most apocalyptic fights. Patrick was always willing to take it further than I was." And then: "If it got to the point where you wanted to put your foot down, there would be no discussion. All of a sudden, out of the blue, 'You can't do that!' We both knew there was no recourse at that point." I was unpredictable and inconsistent when it came to parenting, and I am certain that it was confusing as hell to my kids when everything appeared to be so out of control.

However, I excelled at routine. Schedules and regimens became my saving grace. Benjamin remembers that I "was in charge of meals and the house. Anything that we did on a regular basis, you were awesome at! That's how you built up your repertoire of 'mommying.' Like the procedure of getting us up in the morning, for example. Every moment of the morning was scheduled, consistent, and enforced. We'd get up, get dressed, make our beds, come down and eat breakfast, then wash up and brush our teeth, and be out the door. There was a certain point every night that the kitchen would 'close.' We weren't even allowed to go into the kitchen! Looking back I see that stuff that was routine was the only stuff that really made any sense to you."

This very scheduled, and yet at the same time chaotic, household must have been confusing for Patrick most of the time as well. There is a family story that is told that illustrates this point

suddenly felt the trailer hit the curb and then lurch onto its side and skid to a halt. Benjamin, taking command as he usually did, unzipped the mesh covering and poked his head out. He saw me collapsed on the pavement. "You didn't seem to be hurt, but you were unresponsive. You weren't doing anything, just lying there. I'm pretty sure what happened was that you had one of your 'lightning' episodes. You must have hit the curb and then fallen over. I told Patrick to stay with you and I ran up the driveway to the house we were in front of and asked the lady if I could call 911. Then I went back to sit with Patrick on the curb and wait for the ambulance to come." The paramedics arrived a few minutes later and saw that I had just a few scrapes and bruises. Nothing looked too serious. But when they asked me where I lived, I didn't know. They were alarmed that I appeared so confused, and they held me in the ambulance until I came out of the "lightning" situation and became more coherent. (Remember my old pals "lightning," "piercing headache" and "foggy confusion.")

It was this episode that forced Jim to consider that perhaps not everything was as well with me as he thought. He knew that I might not always be able to find my way home (Hmm . . . because *that's* certainly normal . . .) but he thought that I would always somehow be able to keep the kids safe. This little bike accident forced Jim to rethink. What if I had been in the car? He had no idea that this sort of thing had already occurred while I was driving. He ordered me a medical alert bracelet, which would instruct medical personnel to look in my purse for a card. The card explained that I had suffered from a closed-head injury, that I had memory issues, and that Jim should be telephoned at work if I became incapacitated. A medical alert bracelet seems like a woefully inadequate solution to conceivably hazardous circumstances.

But in his own head, Jim thought that doing *something* concrete, like ordering me a medical alert bracelet, *was* a proper response to his many safety concerns. What else was he to do? He had to be at work, and it wasn't like there was any extra money to hire help for me at home.

Despite my obvious problems, I continued to feign comprehension of the world even among close friends and family. Road trips would invariably trigger "lightning" and confusion. In the summer of 1990, the family drove to Hilton Head, South Carolina, for a weeklong Miller family reunion. I went through the motions well enough so that my brothers, sisters, parents, and grandparents had no idea how little I understood of what was going on. My outward appearance held up well until dinner one night with the entire family in a noisy restaurant. Jim immediately recognized my panicked look and announced that we needed to leave. As we got up, everyone else got up as well. And as I was walking out of the restaurant with Jim and the boys, the rest of the family was right behind us. Jim remembers me looking back and saying, "Who are these people, and why are they following us?"

A photograph taken that week shows the Meck family among the palm trees. Benjamin is staring off in one direction, Patrick in the other. Jim is smiling at the camera, and I am gazing off into nothingness, my eyes unfocused and blank. My sister Barb observed that in that picture, "You looked so lost. You were able to put on a good front, and follow along, and participate in the family activities. But I never understood that you didn't really have a clue of what to do, or what was going on."

With every passing day, there were new struggles, and Jim's temper got shorter and shorter. On the drive back to Baltimore from Hilton Head, our bikes fell off the car and onto the highway.

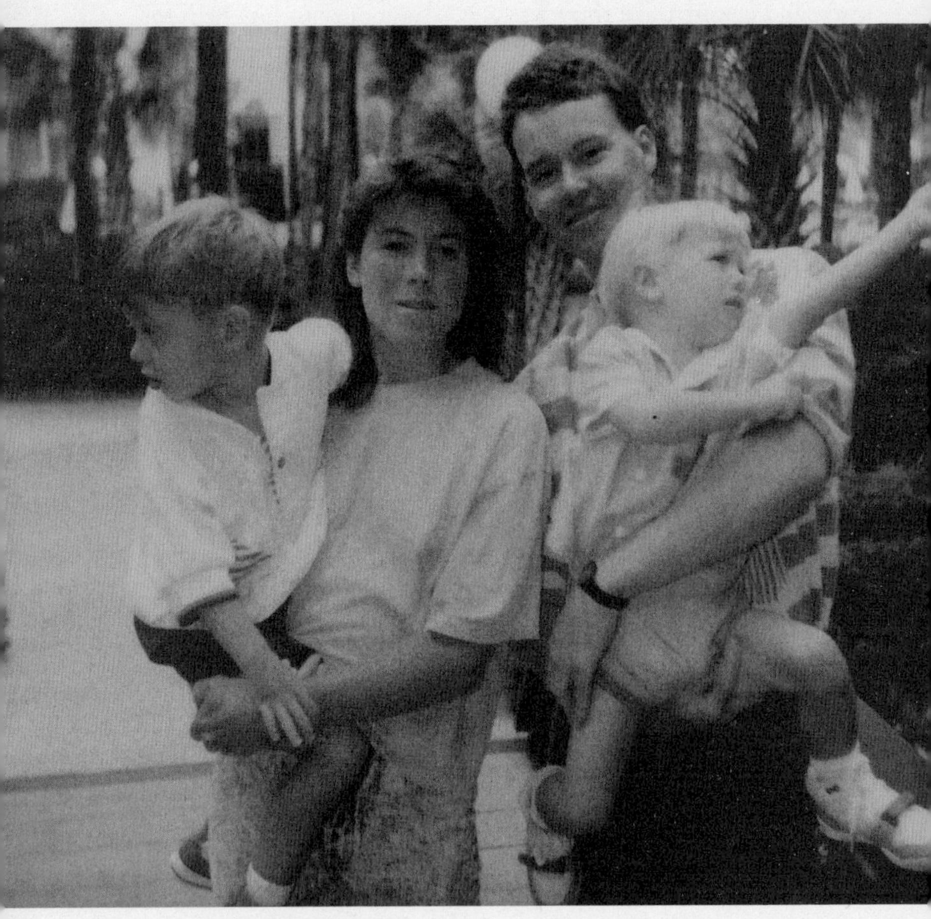

From left: Benjamin, me, Jim, and Patrick. Hilton Head, South Carolina, summer 1990. I look completely out of it.

The straps holding them onto the bike rack had evidently worn down and weakened. They suddenly tore and our bikes went flying off the back of the car and bounced onto the middle of I-95. Jim let out a stream of obscenities and drove recklessly off the highway at the next exit, and then backtracked up the access road. When he got out of the car he told the three of us to "sit there, and shut up!" He then hopped the fence and walked out onto I-95. He held up his hands to stop the traffic, picked up both bikes, carried them to the side of the road, and threw them over the fence. Our bikes were terribly bent and broken, but somehow Jim managed to attach them back onto the bike rack. For a long time afterward, he was really, really angry, so the boys and I just stayed quiet while he drove. I get a sick feeling in my stomach—it actually clenches—even now when I think back to that incident and Jim's fury.

The very next summer, I went with the boys to Florida to visit my sister Barb and her husband, Scott, in Gainesville. I don't know why Jim didn't join us. He may have come along as far as his parents' house in Georgia, and then ended up wanting to spend time with them. During our stay, Barb, Scott, Benjamin, Patrick, and I all drove to Orlando to visit Disney World. It was probably a long, busy, hot, overstimulating day, and that night—ironically enough, during the Electric Light Parade—the "lightning" went off in my head. Barb remembers me grabbing my head and saying, "I don't feel good." And then I checked out. She says I was just gone. I couldn't move. I was paralyzed. I couldn't walk. I was crying because my head hurt terribly. "And we were packed in with thousands of other people watching the parade, Barb says. Somehow, she found me a wheelchair and she and I headed for the car. But she soon discovered that she couldn't take a wheelchair on the monorail—the quieter of the two options—to the parking lot. Instead, we had to go on the large ferryboat, which, Barb recalls, entertained passengers with loud music. She says I could barely talk and I was holding my head in my hands, and people kept coming up and asking if I needed any help. At the hotel the next morning, I was still a mess. Barb can remember checkout time coming and going. She describes me as being "really groggy and slow, almost in slow motion." (There they are again—my trinity—"lightning," "piercing headache," and "foggy confusion.")

Perhaps as a result of that lightning episode, I have no memories of this vacation. In fact, when I was talking to Benjamin recently and he mentioned this trip, I was convinced that he was mistaken. I told him the only time I thought he had ever gone to Disney World was when he went with his high school choir.

I have one final, albeit vague, recollection from our time in Baltimore. I can picture myself sitting on our yellowish easy chair next to the fireplace crying. Then I can remember Jim forcefully loading me into the car, driving me somewhere, and leaving me there. The one clear memory I have regarding this episode is thinking, I can't lose it anymore because Jim gets so pissed off when I do. I am going to have to try harder and do better. Did I take yet another trip to a psych ward? Am I confusing this time with the other time Jim took me to the psychiatric hospital right after we moved to Baltimore when we were staying at the Welcome Inn? I don't know, and Jim doesn't remember, either. But as he comments, "Just because I don't remember, doesn't mean it didn't happen."

11

~

Ode to My Family

—Cranberries

For many years, I was beyond clueless about the whole "marriage and family" concept. I never knew exactly how I was supposed to act around people in the first place, *and* I wasn't sure where I fit into all the words that I heard being thrown around: mom, dad, husband, wife, spouse, son, daughter, brother, sister, son-in-law, daughter-in-law (for some reason I always thought of "in-law" as being like "in jail"), cousin, sibling; dating, engaged, married, pregnant; infant, toddler, teenager, grandma, grandpa, aunt, uncle, related by blood (. . . Ewwww! . . . Blood? . . . Really?!). The list seemed endless.

There were way too many words in the English language to describe relationships among families. I was "Su Meck," but Benjamin and Patrick called me "Mom." I also called the woman who lived in Houston "Mom," but when I sent letters to her I wrote "Mom Miller" on the outside of the envelope, not "Mom Meck." The little boys lived with me, but I didn't live with the woman in Houston, and they called her "Grandma." Benjamin and Patrick were called "brothers," but I had "brothers," too, and Rob and Mark were nothing like Benjamin and Patrick. And my brothers did not live together or with me. I had "sisters," and I was sometimes called a "sister," but Barb and Diane had different last names from me too. If we were related, why did we all have different names? And where were Benjamin and Patrick's sisters? Jim didn't call me "Mom," or "sister," and most of the time he didn't call me "Su." Instead he called me "Subie," or his "wife," and showed me pictures of our "wedding." But where were Benjamin and Patrick in those pictures? And who were all those others in the photos? (Thankfully, only about twenty people attended my wedding.) A big part of the problem was that I continued (for years) to have an incredibly literal mind. To a certain extent, I still do.

So I just did what I always did. I sat back, listened, observed, and tried to make sense out of what people around me said and did. And then I attempted to act like everyone else and to fit in as best as I could, or at least not stick out. If I was mostly quiet, and appeared happy and agreeable, then life was good. I learned to go along to get along, and nobody questioned my behavior. In fact, quite the opposite. Everyone who knew me from before, my family especially, kept telling me how much "nicer," "quieter," "more content," "more pleasant," "calmer," and "more good-natured" I was now. My dad loved to say, jokingly (I think), "We should've hit her over the head with a two-by-four a long time ago!" All of those positive reactions were a good thing, right? I can remember that when I was around, friends and family seemed to smile and laugh a lot. Not that I understood why they did. Or why "quiet and content" was such a good thing. But smiles and laughter are good, right?

But then I would often get even more confused because depending on those in attendance, "nice, pleasant, and calm" did not always equal "right" or "correct." There seemed at times to be different rules with Jim at home as opposed to at church, for instance. I tended to agree with nearly all of Jim's opinions, ideas, and decisions, mostly because I didn't understand what he was talking about the majority of the time and agreeing with him just made life easier. I would literally nod and smile, just like some sort of creepy Stepford wife. And more often than not, he was pleased. But occasionally he would become infuriated with me for *not* arguing with him! Why? Why on earth would someone *want* to yell and argue? He would call me "a doormat," "a scared rabbit," "stupid," and "totally ignorant." And I suppose it was true. (I still am about a lot of things.) But that was because I didn't understand why he wanted me to disagree with him. Wasn't he the one who was supposed to know what was best? He would shout that he wanted me to "offer a fucking opinion for once in your life!" But I couldn't because I honestly didn't have an opinion. About much of anything.

Sex was another thing that baffled me, because "nice" in our bedroom was definitely not "right"! Jim had long since explained the birds and the bees to me. Even so, I had no idea what the hell I was supposed to do, or why. I have vague memories, from when I don't know, of Jim telling me very firmly that we were supposed to have sex because we were married, and that's what married people do. He told me how much he loved me and just wanted to be able to show me. Except when we did eventually engage in sexual activity, I thought it was disgusting, gross, smelly, and sweaty, and it really hurt! Plus, Jim frightened me.

Just like I did not comprehend most of what was going on during the day, nighttime really bewildered me. Jim is not, and has never been as long as I can remember, a quiet sleeper. And I don't just mean that he snores, although he does that, too. No, Jim is "not quiet" in a disturbing, scary way. Certainly not every night, but often enough, he becomes talkative and very physical with me. Despite being asleep, he has shouted at me, and called me all manner of derogatory names, as well as many other women's names. He has slapped and scratched me, held me down, kept a pillow over my face, and hit my head repeatedly against the wall or headboard. Yet what is even more upsetting to me than any of that stuff is the fact that I thought that this behavior was totally normal. And it is troubling that I put up with this craziness for so long thinking it was just part of what "marriage" was. I honestly did not know that I could say "No!" or defend myself in any way. When I finally figured out, after several years, that this conduct maybe wasn't so normal, I asked Jim about it. I think we were living in the house on Beaver Ridge Road, in the Washington suburb of Montgomery Village, at the time. I have no idea what I actually asked him, but probably something like, "Why do you feel the need to occasionally hit me, scratch me, and shout at me during the night?" He probably looked at me as if I was insane. He says he honestly had no recollection of ever doing anything hurtful or hateful to me.

Since then Jim has participated in a number of sleep studies, and has tried various medications, for things like "sleep drunkenness" and a variety of other diagnoses, but unfortunately "Nighttime Jim" has to this day never completely gone away. There seems to be no kind of pattern as to when the "bad nights" will occur, and sometimes up to six months will pass with blissful, uninterrupted sleep. And then those bad nights appear again out of the blue.

Over the years, I have come to learn to love. And I understand the difference now between "loving" ice cream and the "love" I have for my kids. But what about Jim? That is a tricky and far more complicated question. If it makes any sense at all, I have always loved Jim, and I have never loved Jim. In a way, Jim was assigned to me. I never really had a say, which sounds incredibly cruel, but that's essentially the way it is. Jim is all I know. I have only ever made love to one person. I have only ever shared a bedroom, a bathroom, and a bank account with one person. I have only ever slow-danced with one person. Before writing this book, I have only ever told one person my deepest secrets, my most hopeful dreams, and my darkest fears. And that person was always Jim. Jim is the only person who has ever made me feel truly beautiful, sexy, and desirable. Even during those times when I am feeling neither beautiful nor sexy, and those other times when I am clearly not desirable. There can be no stronger love anywhere than the love I feel from him at those times. Regrettably, Jim is also the one person who can with no more than a look, a word, or tone of voice make me feel small, scared, stupid, insignificant, embarrassed, and worthless. Bottom line: I have always been trying, and probably will always try, to get Jim's approval, because there is nothing on this earth better. However, there is a conflicting side to his personality, and when that side comes out there is without fail hell to pay! That being said, I am somewhat convinced that his behavior, both good and bad, over the years is directly linked to how much our lives were altered by a ceiling fan when we were both so young.

~

Despite all of this, the Meck family continued to muddle through as best as we could. Even though Jim lost his job in Baltimore early in January of 1991, he thankfully was able to find another job within a few months working for a small software company based outside Boston but with offices in Greenbelt, MD. This job required him to travel most of the time, either to the company's headquarters or around the country selling the company's software. With this new job he was gone for about three weeks out of every month, and even when he was "home," he spent most of his time driving to his office in Maryland, near Washington, D.C., sometimes a two-hour drive one way. Having him away so much was both a blessing and a curse. On the one hand, I was nervous about being by myself with the boys. Jim, regardless of his behavior toward me, was my touchstone. He was familiar and I somehow understood myself better when he was around. On the other hand, I was guaranteed a good night's sleep without Jim, and Benjamin and Patrick's behavior seemed to improve when he was gone. After several months of all this driving and traveling, it became clear that we couldn't stay in Bel Air. Jim decided we would move to Montgomery County, relocating from suburban Baltimore to suburban Washington, to be closer to his office as well as National Airport.

Montgomery Village is a planned community, and a great place to be a young family. There are swimming pools, recreation centers with all kinds of year-round activities and camps for kids, lakes with walking trails and bike paths, and shopping centers all close by. Our house was at the end of a court, and behind it was a little creek and woods to explore.

Jim was away traveling the day the boys and I actually moved into the house on Beaver Ridge Road, and one specific episode from the day is extremely vivid in my mind. This house had a ridiculously dramatic, sweeping two-story foyer with a little balcony right off the master bedroom that looked down over that foyer. (Picture the pope looking down from such a balcony and blessing thousands of devoted Catholic pilgrims inside my front hall.) It did not take long for my boys to come up with a magnificent plan to make this boring moving day into something a bit more exciting. They walked around the house gathering up all the bedding, blankets, towels, linens, sleeping bags, and pillows that they could find and proceeded to build a huge "nest" in that front hall. What was I doing while they were being so industrious? I honestly have no idea. What I do remember is coming upon my five-year-old, thrill-seeking son flying through the air from the balcony, landing (mostly) in the "nest" of bedding, immediately standing up, and beckoning up to his three-year-old brother, who was himself perched on the edge ready to jump! I'm sure my shrieks were heard throughout the neighborhood, but fortunately they did not startle Patrick enough to make him fall. After that incident, I distinctly remember that I literally tied both boys to my physical person for the rest of that day.

Regardless of that shaky start, we settled into our life in Montgomery County. Starting that September, Benjamin attended afternoon kindergarten at Goshen Elementary School, and Patrick was enrolled in the nearby afternoon preschool. At one point I remember Patrick's teacher taking me aside and asking if everything was all right with Jim and me. I nodded and asked why she wanted to know. She said that Patrick told her that his daddy only ever came home to mow the lawn. About this same time, both boys had drawn pictures in their Sunday school classes at Gaithersburg

Presbyterian that included a smiling mom and two smiling boys. No father anywhere in either picture. (Hmm.)

I got another part-time job teaching aerobics classes at Athletic Express, a large gym not far from where we lived. From connections I made working there, I was invited to teach classes at two other gyms, Philbin's and Fitness First. "Part-time" eventually swelled into teaching up to fifteen or sixteen classes a week, with many often back-to-back.

I continued to keep a detailed calendar listing everything I needed to do, and I referred to it several dozen times a day. As long as I was teaching classes, getting Benjamin and Patrick to and from school, driving them to soccer, gymnastics, cherub choir, and dance classes, "helping" with homework and school projects, "volunteering" at the library at the elementary school, preparing meals, doing laundry, going grocery shopping, and cleaning the house, I never had to interact with people at anything more than a superficial level. I came in contact with a lot of people during my days, but didn't, for the most part, know anybody's name and often didn't recognize people from one day to the next. I could play the part of the "Montgomery County Mother" at the kids' schools, and I could turn on the charm to teach aerobics classes, but I was horribly insecure and nervous whenever I had to speak or socialize with anybody for any length of time. I actually *was* only playing the part of a mom. I didn't do things because I *knew* they were the right things to do. I did things because I saw what other moms were doing, and I simply copied what they did. At the health clubs where I worked, it wasn't much different. I initially just copied what other instructors were doing, and over time teaching certain classes became second nature. Eventually, after many years of teaching, I developed my own style and became a fairly popular instructor.

~

Jim and I continued to play the part of a married couple, and eventually we even resumed a sort of sex life. But Jim thinks that sex, from this point on, was simply one of the many things that I just accepted, without question, as part of the marriage and family routine. Now I wash dishes. Now I cook dinner. Now we go to church. Now we have sex. Now I fold the laundry.

He is probably right about that and about me to a certain extent, especially in the beginning. But I can also remember (eventually) countless special times that we shared over our years together, moments that included laughter, passion, intimacy, and a closeness that I have never experienced with anybody else. And I certainly can't remember him ever complaining to me about our sexual escapades, particularly once I finally figured everything out.

But I am jumping ahead.

Early in the fall of 1991, Jim and I received an invitation to attend the wedding ceremony of Kathy VanSchaick and Randy Brown. Kathy was one of the few people that I had kept in touch with from high school and to this day is one of my very best friends. Jim remembers that she was a terrific help to me after my injury, especially after we moved east from Texas, patiently retelling me stories and showing me photos of our high school antics. Kathy and Randy's wedding was to be held in November at Wayne Presbyterian Church, the church I had attended with my own family when we lived outside of Philadelphia. Kathy told me that she and I had been active in choir and youth group at Wayne Presbyterian when we were in high school, and my sister Diane and her husband, Paul, had been married there in 1985.

Philadelphia was an easy drive from Maryland, so it was decided that Jim and I would go to the wedding, but we would leave Benjamin and Patrick with friends for the weekend. I have a feeling that Jim thought (correctly) that attending Kathy's wedding would be stressful enough for me without adding our active four- and five-year-old to the festivities. There would not only be lots of people and confusion, which, in and of itself, could be problematic for me, but also many other guests who most likely would know me from before my injury. They would know me, but I wouldn't have a clue who they were, which was always a bit awkward for everyone.

The sanctuary of Wayne Presbyterian Church is an enormous and gorgeous old stone building, which that Saturday afternoon was made even more beautiful with abundant flower arrangements and other tasteful trimmings. Kathy was gorgeous as well, although I do think she told me she wore white Keds rather than heels. Randy was in his dress uniform from the U.S. Army, looking incredibly handsome. The ceremony itself was not long, but I remember coming to a significant realization as I listened to the pastor speak, and as I listened to Randy and Kathy exchange their vows. *This* is a wedding. After *this* wedding ceremony, Kathy and Randy will be *married* to each other, just like Jim and I are married to each other. I do not have any idea why I made this particular connection on this particular day, but I did, and it has stuck with me as one of my big aha moments. The rest of that day is a blur. I think the reception was right next door at a beautiful old Victorian mansion. I recall a ton of people there, with food, music, drinking, and dancing. But the only thing I *really* remember about that day was thinking constantly, I am *married* to Jim just like Kathy and Randy are married to each other now! This was a strange realization.

That night, back at our hotel room, is the first time I can actually remember enjoying (and better understanding) sex with Jim. And that memory is all the sweeter because I am certain that my beautiful daughter, Kassidy, was conceived that very night.

12

Sweet Child of Mine

—Guns N' Roses

The first thing I did when I found out I was pregnant in the late fall or early winter of 1991 was panic! Panic was followed immediately by a longtime state of denial. I would not have even realized I was pregnant if it wasn't for my friend Jodi. Patrick took gymnastics classes with Jodi's girls at Hills Gymnastics Center, and one morning, while we watched the kids tumble, viewing them through the glass between the parents' waiting area and the gym, Jodi started complaining about how bad her cramps were. I said something like, "I would rather have cramps than be throwing up all the time." She asked me what I meant by that, and I said, "Well, I haven't had a period for a really long time, but I throw up all the time." She gave me her classic incredulous Jodi look, and asked me, "Well? Are you pregnant?" Jodi has never been one to mince words or hold back anything she thinks. She is without filter! When the gymnastics class ended, Jodi insisted we pile all the kids into her mother's Range Rover so her mom could take them all to their house to have lunch and to play. Jodi then took me to Drug Emporium and bought me a pregnancy test kit. We went to my house and she waited while I peed on the stick. Before I even flushed, the "+" was showing. Holy shit! Now what? Initially I thought, Gross! There's someone living and growing *inside* of me! What did I know about being pregnant? Nothing. What did I know about giving birth to babies? Nothing. What did I know about taking care of newborn babies? Nothing. Was this something that would just go away if ignored? Maybe. Possibly.

Jim continued to travel. For the most part he remained gone for three weeks out of every month, so it was no surprise that he was away the week I found out I was pregnant. Even when he came home for the weekend, I didn't know how or what to tell him. I didn't know what to do at all. I never went to the doctor. I didn't even know who my doctor was or where he or she was even located. A couple of weeks passed before Jim asked if I was okay. I came down one morning while he was making his coffee, and I barely made it to the bathroom before throwing up. I told him right then that I was pregnant (and also how much I hated the smell of his coffee). He was over-the-moon excited about the news! That day at work, he looked up Ob-gyns in Montgomery Village that would take our health insurance and, thankfully, he found Dr. Brockett Muir.

Dr. Muir was the perfect fit because he was the quintessential old-school obstetrician. By 1991, when I first met him, he seemingly had successfully delivered half of the population of

Montgomery County under the age of thirty-five. He didn't get outwardly excited, flustered, nervous, or worried about much of anything, and he always took tons of time answering my endless questions in his office, as he sat fingering his packet of Camels. He was a no-nonsense, straight-talking guy, with compassion and heart. Dr. Muir was the first (and probably to this day the *only*) doctor, other than my kids' pediatricians and their dentist, that I fully trusted, respected, and liked.

Even so, I was so afraid of what another baby would mean for our family. By the fall of 1991, Benjamin was five, and in kindergarten, and Patrick was four, and in preschool. They both knew how to walk, talk, dress themselves, go potty (in the potty), blow their own noses, eat with silverware, and drink from a glass. And most of the time, I could do all that stuff, too. But a baby wouldn't know how to do anything, and it would depend on me to do everything for it. That was a terrifying thought! Would Benjamin be able to help me with this like he helped out with everything else? I was unclear as to whether he could. The three of us, the boys and I, worked well together as a trio. Sure, there were bad moments. If truth be told, a *lot* of bad moments. And I was exhausted most of the time. But Benjamin, Patrick, and I got through most days without too many life-altering catastrophes. How would a new baby change the system that we had in place? Granted, it was a loose and vague system, but it was a system that seemed to work for us.

Would I still be able to teach aerobics? I was working at a few different health clubs now, teaching at least twelve classes a week. But I also was thinking about branching out into personal training. Several people had approached me about training them one-on-one, and I was seriously considering the idea. The notion of having to give up my classes, and the paychecks that went along with them, was not a happy one. Jim and I barely made ends meet as it was. Sometimes we didn't, and when that happened there was a lot of putting up with Jim's shouting and carrying on. Would a new baby leave us utterly destitute? And what about the time factor? How much time did a new baby take? I didn't have any extra time in my day, so how exactly would that work? Would Jim know what to do? Would he ever be around at all to help out?

I started watching women with babies in the grocery store, in the neighborhood, at church, at the gyms where I worked, at Goshen Elementary when I picked up Benjamin after school, and at the Montgomery Village preschool where Patrick went. Babies could be cute, but they seemed like a lot of work. They couldn't be left alone for a second, even if they were in a car seat or a stroller. Most babies also seemed really messy to me. They drooled, they coughed, spitup, and their noses always seemed to be running, which was really gross. Putting a coat, or a sweater, or shoes, or boots, or mittens on a baby looked incredibly difficult and complicated. Babies were fussy and squirmy, and their movements were so random. Even holding them seemed to be a struggle.

But then at one of my early appointments with Dr. Muir, I heard my baby's heartbeat. Almost instantly I was in love. I suddenly had an entirely new outlook about this little being inside of me. Pregnancy didn't seem quite so gross and disgusting to me anymore, and the whole "birth" part was so far away anyway that I didn't even worry about that. I had absolutely no appreciation for, or understanding of, what was to come. Suddenly I started seeing moms out with their babies in a whole different way. Moms didn't seem quite so frazzled, and babies didn't seem quite so grubby. I began to really pay attention to everything I ate, and I drank gallons of milk. I continued to teach my aerobics classes with

Dr. Muir's blessing: "Su, your body would go into shock if you stopped doing any of that exercising. By all means, keep up with the activities that you're used to doing."

Other than throwing up pretty much all the time until February or so, my pregnancy proceeded without too much difficulty. I can remember coming out of a monthly appointment with Dr. Muir close to Valentine's Day and smelling doughnuts. Montgomery Donuts had a shop right across the street from the medical office complex, and I *needed* doughnuts. I told myself, I'll surprise the boys and take doughnuts home for their after-school snack. I bought two heart-shaped doughnuts with pink- and red-colored sprinkles, and eleven jelly doughnuts, for an even baker's dozen. Every single one of those jelly doughnuts was gone by the time I picked up Benjamin and Patrick from school that afternoon. They were both excited about getting a special after-school snack, and when Patrick asked where my doughnut was, I just said, "Mommy already ate hers." I always blamed Montgomery Donuts for the more than fifty pounds. I gained during my pregnancy with Kassidy. When it came to jelly doughnuts, I had absolutely no willpower whatsoever.

In March of 1992, Jim decided to take Benjamin; Patrick; my brother Mark; and his then girlfriend, Tiffany and me skiing in Snowshoe, West Virginia. Mark and Tiffany were both undergraduate students at James Madison University, and they had a weeklong spring break in mid-March. I checked with Dr. Muir to make sure that skiing would be a sanctioned activity for me, as I was now well into my second trimester. He did not seem the least bit worried about the baby, or me, and sent me on my way, telling me to relax and have a good time.

Snowshoe was a blast. We arrived the first night in an actual

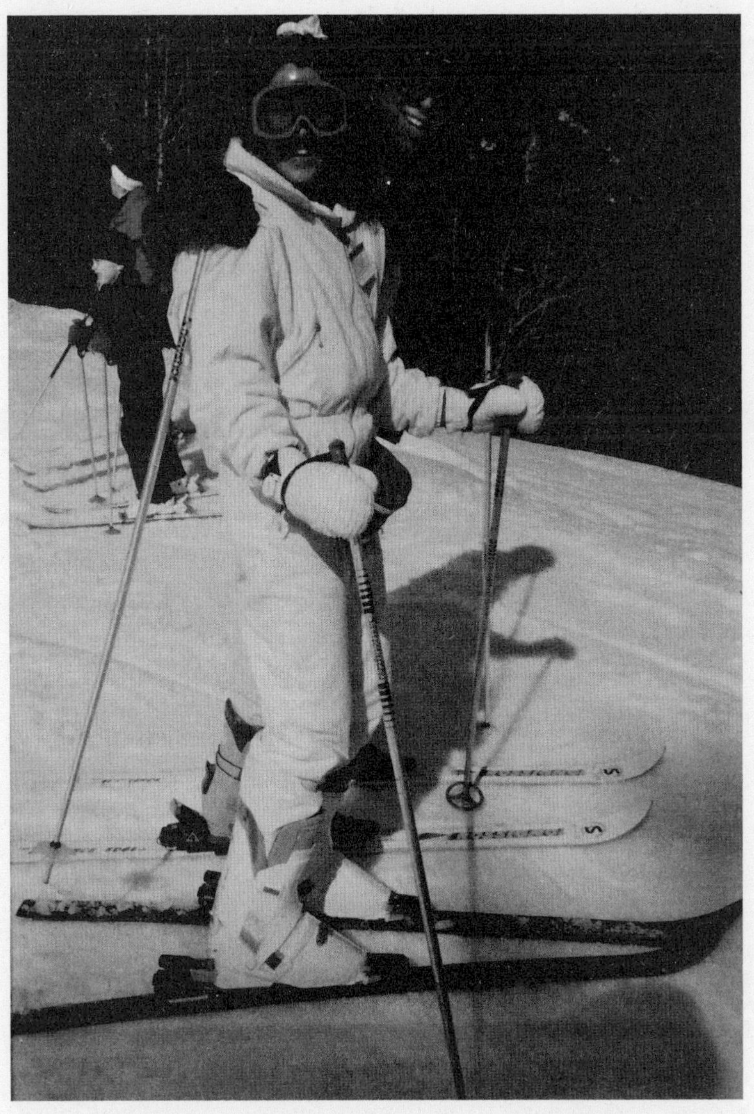

My brother Mark and me at Snowshoe, West Virginia,
in March 1992. I am almost six months pregnant with Kassidy.

blizzard, which was a little scary as we drove on unfamiliar roads up the mountain to the resort. However, because so much snow fell that first night, the ski conditions were glorious the entire time we were there, and because it was late in the season, it was not the least bit crowded. The boys, who were only four and five, learned to ski, went sledding, built snow castles, and sipped hot chocolate. I had never been skiing before, and it had been a while since Mark, Tiffany, and Jim had been on skis. But they picked it back up quickly, and pretty soon all three were off looking for more dangerous mountains to conquer. I was happy going up and down the bunny hill by myself with my skis in a snowplow position for the entire first day. However, I got more adventurous by day three, and even attempted a few longer and steeper blue square trails. This trip was by far the best vacation, and I think the only vacation, that we ever took as a family that was purely just for the fun of it. In fact, I still have my Snowshoe sweatshirt that I purchased that week. I just cannot bring myself to part with it.

We had only been home from that perfect family vacation for a few weeks before my pregnancy took a turn for the worse.

~

Early in April, Benjamin's kindergarten class began learning about all the ways that five- and six-year-olds can help save their planet. These discussions were most likely leading up to some kind of culminating Earth Day activity at the school. April wasn't always especially warm, but by this point in the year the slightest bit of sunshine would drive us all outside for some "fresh air." On this particular day, Patrick, Benjamin, and I had decided to take a walk around Lake Marion, near our home, before supper. At the last moment they both decided they wanted to ride their bikes instead. I said fine, as long as they followed the walking-Mommy bike rules. Basically, they were not allowed to ride their bikes so far ahead of me that I couldn't see them and they couldn't see me. They had to stop and wait (patiently, without whining) for me to catch up. They both agreed, and we were off. When I arrived at the top of the path that led down to Lake Marion, they were waiting for me. Patrick asked if they could ride all around the lake without stopping. I said yes, and they were off like a shot. I started walking around the lake, watching the boys as they sped ahead. I can remember thinking how amazed I was at how quickly Patrick had picked up riding a two-wheeler. They rode up behind me and I remember pretending to be shocked and amazed at how fast they both rode. They asked if they could go around again, and we all laughed and recited together the words from Dr. Seuss's *Go, Dog. Go!* "The dogs are all going around and around. Go around again!" And once again, they sped off.

A few moments later, I saw that the bikes had both been abandoned on the path. I then saw Patrick standing next to a tree near the lake. He waved at me. As I got closer, I heard a big splash. Patrick turned and ran toward me, screaming, "Benjamin just fell in the lake!" I rushed forward through all the weeds and brambles. I can remember spotting Benjamin's jean jacket with the navy-blue sleeves and hood. Without thinking at all, I stepped into the icy water, grabbed for that hood, and pulled as hard as I could. I lost my balance with the first pull and fell deeper into the water, but I was closer now to where Benjamin was, so I got a better hold on him and pulled again, as hard as I could. That time I got him and literally threw him up on the bank of the lake. I knew that both Benjamin and Patrick were crying, but I couldn't move toward them at first. I was in so much *pain!* And when I looked down, there was blood. Somehow, I got myself out of the lake and got the boys back on their bikes. Benjamin was babbling this whole time about "a plastic milk jug hurting the earth!" But I wasn't really listening to him. He was soaking wet and shivering uncontrollably. I was unsure whether or not he would be able to ride his bike. I was shivering and wet as well, but I was more concerned about the pain and all the blood. I just wanted to sit down, curl up in a ball, and go to sleep, but something gave me the strength to walk home, encouraging the boys the whole time, saying over and over, "Everything is fine. Everyone is fine."

This is what Benjamin remembers about that fateful day: "I fell through the thin ice of the lake and I was in the frigid water. And you immediately jumped in. You might have thrown Patrick out of the way first, or in the other direction into the grass and then jumped in after me. I remember that you waded into the lake and just bodily grabbed me up and then you ran back so now we're both soaking wet and freezing. So freezing cold. And then we just ran home. I was shivering my ass off! We went inside and you went and got towels and blankets and wrapped me up cinnamon-bun style in all those towels and blankets, and you laid down and had me call someone. I don't know if the cold shock of the water immediately sent you into labor. I just remember you screaming, making these horrible noises of anguish. And I remember you expressing pain in your face and verbally and me asking if you were all right, and you repeating, 'It's all right, it's the baby, it's the baby.' I'm fuzzy as to who took us to the hospital or when Dad came. I think back to my childhood, there were more days that he wasn't home than there were days that he was home. I've got to believe that it was me calling 911. Both Patrick and I, just given our situation, we did routine drills on, Where is all the stuff we need in the house? How do you dial 911? How do you talk to the operator? We had a phone list on the refrigerator. I was only six, and this was the second or third time I had called 911 on your behalf."

The situation was clearly a serious one. Jim says, "I don't remember how I got to the hospital, either. I recall sitting in a conference room in Waltham, Mass., being interrupted for a phone call and someone telling me that you'd had an accident. The next memory I have is being by your side in the ER at Shady Grove Hospital. At the hospital the doctor told me that your uterus might 'tear itself apart.' You were only at twenty-three or twenty-four weeks of gestation; your uterus was weakened by two previous cesarean deliveries, the first of which had been an emergency, and therefore a vertical rather than horizontal incision. You were not supposed to go into labor with this pregnancy. You had lost a lot of blood, and your condition was deemed too delicate for a helicopter ride, so they hurriedly bundled you in an ambulance and rushed you to Georgetown Medical Center downtown. The doctors couldn't understand why you knew none of your own medical history. You bluffed and said I kept track of all that and I just automatically covered for you."

A young resident at Georgetown examined me and delivered an unexpected ultimatum: "There's two ways we can go here. We can do what we can to save the child, or you can decide to do whatever needs to be done to help the mother. If you opt to improve the mother's condition, we can't do that here." Georgetown University Hospital was a Catholic hospital, sworn to protect our baby at any cost. The resident explained to Jim that I had suffered an abruption, in which the placenta was partially torn away from my uterine wall, and that I had lost, and continued to lose, quite a bit of blood. The doctor gave us five minutes. Jim recalls, "For me, it was like a flashback to that moment at the other hospital in Fort Worth: 'Bring your sons and tell your wife good-bye.' I didn't need five minutes. I told the doctors to save the baby because that was going to be the only way anyone at that hospital would dispense *any* treatment to you." They administered large doses of magnesium sulfate to me, meant to slow the contractions. It was initially too much. My vital signs flickered. Jim summoned the head nurse, who reduced the dosage. Fortunately, my body eventually stabilized somewhat, but the contractions never stopped.

I spent almost a week in the hospital, and when I was released it was with strict orders to stay in bed. Jim talked with my parents and it was decided that my mom would come up and stay with us and help with the boys as well as meals and housework so I wouldn't feel compelled to do anything. I was once again baffling the medical community by somehow holding on to Kassidy through three months of constant labor.

On July 13, 1992, Kassidy Taylor Meck was delivered by cesarean section. My sister Barb wrote in her journal a few days later: "7-18-92: Su and Kassidy went home yesterday and all is going well. Su sounded so upbeat and happy. She feels better than she has for months. They are already more like best friends than they are mother and daughter."

~

Dr. Muir is a big reason why I held on to Kassidy until the middle of July. He kept telling me, "Your daughter is in the best possible place"—inside me—"and the longer you can hold on to her the better she will be in the long run. You can either have a few months of discomfort now, or there is a possibility that she will suffer a lifetime of discomfort if she is born too early." The first time I saw her, just like when I first heard her heartbeat, I fell head over heels in love with her. I was terrified that I was going to break her somehow, and I worried constantly about whether she was feeling too warm or too cold, or if she was hungry or sleepy. I didn't know who to ask how I was supposed to hold her, or how I was supposed to know what she wanted. Because I had two young boys, everybody just assumed I was an old pro and knew exactly what to do.

I remember Jim bringing Benjamin and Patrick to visit their new sister and me in the hospital. Benjamin wanted to read her a book, and so he brought Dr. Seuss's *Marvin K. Mooney, Will You Please Go Now!* from home. He sat and read that book particularly loudly to Kassidy and Patrick. He was so loud as he read, and so close to her (so she could see all the pictures), I thought for sure that Kassidy would be afraid and start to cry, but surprisingly, she didn't.

I can remember holding Kassidy and just staring at her. She had, and still has, these huge, gorgeous blue eyes. I was scared to death that I was going to hurt her because I didn't know what I was doing, and I desperately didn't want to do anything wrong.

Benjamin says he remembers the day that Kassidy came home. "Kassidy was asleep in her baby carrier and you just set her right down on the family room floor. It's so strange to think back to when she was so tiny. I know that some of the memories that I have of Kassidy as a baby and toddler are kind of secondary memories from pictures I have seen, or stories that you tell. But I can remember both Patrick and me looking at her and then each other and thinking, 'We don't want to deal with this.' And so we played outside a lot more often. When Kassidy cried it was really loud, and you would just drop whatever you were doing and rush to her immediately. I can remember it taking you like more than ten minutes to change Kassidy's diaper. You were with her pretty much all the time. Kassidy nursed until she was almost five, which was probably excessive. And maybe because of that, you two were always together. Even now, you're more like sisters than mother and daughter."

It's true that the dynamics of our family were fairly unusual. Kassidy and I never had a typical mother-daughter relationship. We always seemed kind of on a different wavelength than most other mothers and daughters. I was just beginning to learn how to learn as Kassidy came into my life. Benjamin and Patrick's job in the family was to look out for us. Then there was Jim, who was always really far away, traveling for work.

I probably did devote much more time to Kassidy, at least initially, than I did to anyone or anything else. To some extent, I just didn't know when to stop. Exactly how much care was enough for a completely helpless baby? Patrick and Benjamin, and even Jim, probably felt a bit neglected, and in all likelihood they felt a bit resentful of Kassidy at first. But I couldn't help myself. Kassidy became my everything in the summer of 1992. She was my happy, healthy, perfect baby girl. And she and I, in a sense, ended up growing up together.

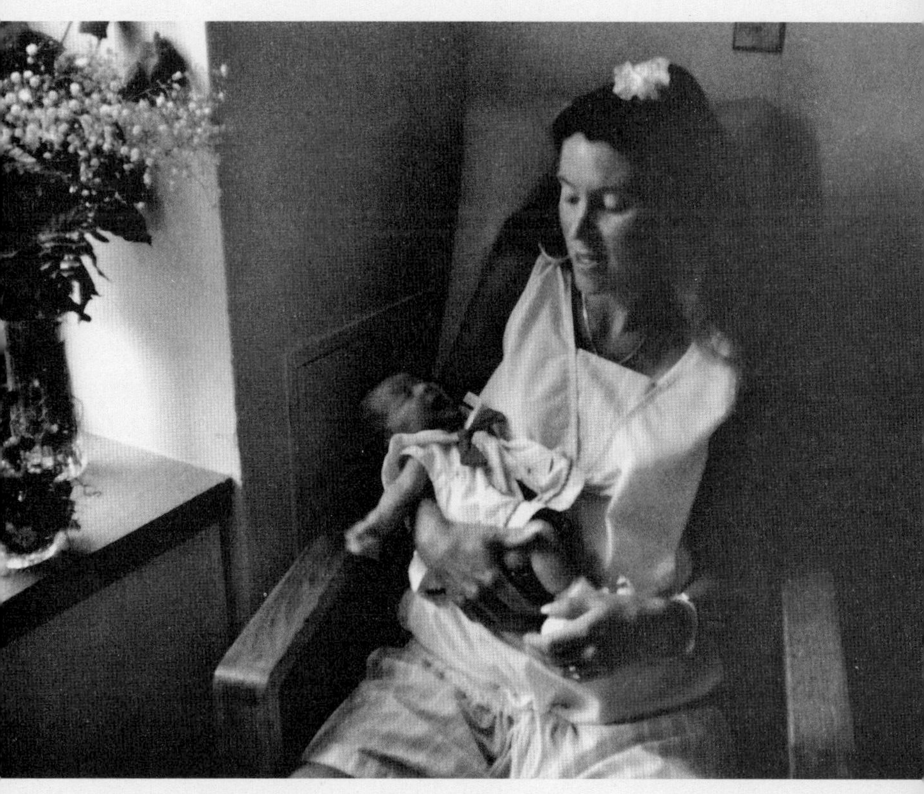

Right before leaving the hospital with Kassidy
in July 1992. I was a nervous wreck!

13

School

—Supertramp

After Kassidy was born, Jim went back to his life of traveling. He was now working for a management consulting firm in northern Virginia and his territory was "the world." So instead of just being away for days or weeks, he would be gone sometimes for months at a time. Sure, they paid well, but Jim essentially sold his soul in order to work there. This particular company made the fictional company in John Grisham's book *The Firm* look like a friggin' preschool. I rarely knew where he was. Jim never left us itineraries, and I didn't know enough to ask for one each time he left. And I probably would not have been able to read them even if he did. He would occasionally call from wherever he was, but often the difference in time was puzzling to me. How was it that he could be getting ready to go out to dinner if I was just getting the boys their breakfast? How was it he was telling me good night right as I was coming home after teaching my morning aerobics classes?

As Jim traveled the globe, I would like very much to say that Benjamin, Patrick, Kassidy, and I led an idyllic life in Montgomery County, keeping the home fires burning, so to speak, awaiting the arrival of our man of the house. In reality, the kids and I continued to lead a chaotic life, with six-year-old Benjamin and now even five-year-old Patrick acting as the men of the house. I was getting better at remembering what needed to be done, as long as I had my huge stickered calendar. Meals were kept simple, and occasionally forgotten. Having a baby, even a baby as easy as Kassidy, still took its toll on all of us. We continued to play the "What are we doing today?" game each morning and I think that helped. The boys can remember me having a lot of "lightning," and even though my episodes didn't faze them, I still can't imagine what could have happened during those times when I was all but incapacitated. Scary.

That fall Benjamin started first grade, and Patrick was enrolled in afternoon kindergarten at Goshen. Fortunately, the school was close enough that I could put Kassidy in a stroller and walk to get both guys in the afternoons. Mostly I remembered. If I didn't, Benjamin waited for Patrick's teacher to bring out the kindergartners, got Patrick, and they walked home together. No biggie, right?

Benjamin started getting "homework" in first grade, so my formal education started about that time as well. Benjamin and I learned to spell *fan, man, ten, pen,* and *land* together. Another week we learned *win, thin, on, pond,* and *spin.* On and on we went. Every week there were new words to learn and spell. I did all the activities with Benjamin. He helped me with ABC order on Mondays, and we would come up with silly sentences together on Tuesdays. On Wednesdays, we wrote each spelling word out five times. Boring. The test was always on Friday, so Thursday nights at bedtime we would quiz each other. Even Patrick, by this time of the week, knew how to read and spell all Benjamin's spelling words.

I got a job volunteering in the Goshen Elementary School library one afternoon each week. I took Kassidy with me. Kassidy had the ability to charm everyone around her with her blue eyes, her bright smile, and her happy disposition, so it was seldom a problem. She sat quietly (most days) while I shelved books. In truth, I never did much shelving. Instead, I sat in the stacks with Kassidy and tried to read, looking at the pictures in those children's books and picking out words I had learned from Benjamin's, and eventually Patrick's, spelling lists.

In math, Benjamin was learning addition and later in the year subtraction. We bought flash cards and took turns coaching each other. Again Patrick learned his addition and subtraction facts right along with us. I'm thinking now that Patrick must have been really bored the following year in first grade.

I suppose I am making this sound far too simple. Picture the cozy kitchen with Kassidy asleep on my shoulder as we are all sitting around the kitchen table. Benjamin and Patrick sitting quietly eating their after-school snack while dutifully working on their assignments from school. Then picture the exact opposite, and *that* might be a bit closer to the way it really was. Kassidy had to be awakened from a nap to be put in her stroller and taken out in the cold so we could pick up her brothers from school. She was sometimes whiny and hungry. Benjamin and Patrick were thinking that the last thing they wanted to do, after being cooped up in school all day, was sit down and do homework. They just wanted to play. But if I had to teach a class that evening, they would have to come with me to the health club nursery. Or if they had dance class, gymnastics, or choir, then homework had to be done first thing or it would be forgotten altogether. Nobody was happy with this arrangement. Benjamin had the attention span of a chipmunk when it came to school work, and I constantly had to bring him back to the task at hand. Patrick got bored easily and wanted my undivided attention. Duh! He was FIVE!

Many afternoons all this homework business ended in tears and/or shouting, with homework simply left unfinished. Sometimes I would try to write a note to Benjamin's first-grade teacher, to explain that he understood the concept of the math work sheet, but was only able to complete five of the twenty-five problems. She probably thought Benjamin had written the note himself.

In November, I was assigned a thirty-minute time slot to have a conference with Benjamin's teacher. I was nervous. This was something new, and I didn't know what to expect. Benjamin was not allowed to go with me. I don't remember having Kassidy with me, either. Did I leave her at home with the boys? I must have. When I got to the school, I walked to Benjamin's classroom and I stood awkwardly in the doorway until the teacher acknowledged me. She took a thick folder off the top of a large stack of thick folders and invited me in. She showed me to Benjamin's desk and looked at me. I looked back at her. After a few seconds of uncomfortable silence, she said, "Please have a seat." Where? On Benjamin's tiny chair? At his tiny desk? She sat down on another tiny chair, so I sat down, too. She asked if Mr. Meck would be joining me. I almost laughed out loud. And sitting on these tiny chairs?

No way! I couldn't even picture Jim in this classroom. I said I didn't think so because he was in Thailand. She looked at me again and then continued (this is an approximate conversation):

Teacher: Please look in Benjamin's desk.

Me: (Looking in Benjamin's desk.) It's kind of messy.

Teacher: Yes. It is. And that's after I had him stay in from recess yesterday so he could clean it.

Me: Oh.

Teacher: He did not clean it. He sat in here and ground up almost all of my colored chalk instead. He made a terrible mess.

Me: I'm sorry. (I didn't know what I was supposed to say. This was even more difficult than I imagined it would be.)

Teacher: In fact, Benjamin rarely does what he is told to do. He does not sit in his seat properly. He bothers all of the other children. I've had to move his desk four times this year and it's only November. He sings constantly. He has a smart mouth and sometimes talks back. He does not ever complete his seat work. He has a terrible time staying on task. I fear he won't learn to read this year, because he has appalling attention problems. I've never seen such dreadful attention problems in any other six-year-old. Ever. His handwriting is atrocious. He doesn't even seem to care or try. I think we need to get him on some sort of work contract right away.

(I just sat there in stunned silence. Should I be writing any of this down? I didn't understand half the words she was saying, so I think I may have sort of tuned her out until she came back with:)

Teacher: So, Mrs. Meck, what do you think? What should be done?

Me: Um.

Teacher: I think a work contract is the first step to getting Benjamin back on track. He's obviously a bright little boy. He has an amazing vocabulary for someone his age. But he needs direction. He needs focus. He needs discipline. Is there a place and time he always does his homework at home?

Me: (I thought of the craziness that was "homework time.") Yes.

Teacher: Because I noticed that his homework is rarely completed. Do you check his homework?

Me: (I thought of Benjamin and me doing our spelling words in ABC order together.) Yes.

Teacher: And I'm sure you have noticed that it is often not completed.

Me: Yes. There's not always time.

Teacher: I know there is a new baby at your house. Benjamin always talks about Kassidy. Benjamin always talks. I understand it must be difficult for you, but please try to make sure he does his homework every night. It's best for him to form good habits for schoolwork at this stage of the game. I'm sure you understand. Thank you for coming.

I didn't understand at all but I was dismissed as another mom and dad entered the room together. Benjamin's teacher walked to her desk, set down Benjamin's folder, and picked the next one from the top of the pile. I left, went home, hugged Benjamin, and cried.

Benjamin's school days never got much better after first grade. He struggled with everything associated with school all the way through high school. He hated going. He hated doing homework. He loved to read, once he finally learned, but hated to write. He didn't make friends easily, but didn't seem to care too much about that, either. Outside of the classroom he was intelligent, curious, inquisitive, very funny, and perceptive. There is no doubt he was a handful. He was much smarter than I was at a very early age, and could talk his way into and out of anything. He began to be a compulsive liar, but the stories he told were often funny and sort of interesting.

His third-grade teacher was a nightmare for him. She told me at his conference that November that Benjamin still was not reading because of his horrifying attention issues. She said that I would continue to hold him back if I didn't consider putting him on Ritalin. I certainly didn't want to hold him back, so I spoke to Benjamin's pediatrician, and he started Benjamin on a moderate dose of Ritalin soon after Thanksgiving. And Benjamin did show marked improvement in school after that. He was reading within the month, and not simple chapter books, either. He skipped them altogether and went right to the Boxcar Children series by Gertrude Chandler Warner. He then moved quickly to the Madelene L'Engle books like *A Wrinkle in Time* that Santa brought him that year for Christmas.

Hooray! Benjamin was reading! Except now he was constantly getting in trouble for hiding books in his desk and reading them when he was supposed to be paying attention to social studies or some other such "nonsense" according to Benjamin. I kind of agreed. Everyone had been so concerned about his learning to read, and then it seemed like he got in trouble for reading. I did not understand.

Eventually, Patrick started taking Ritalin as well, and homework got a bit easier in the afternoons. Not easy, but some days, easier. Both boys had daily homework by then, which was always fun. (Not.) Kassidy was two. That was fun, too. (Still not.) I continued to teach aerobics classes. Jim continued to travel. I got good at making excuses for him and why he wasn't ever at concerts, recitals, games, and back-to-school nights. I don't remember being sad or resentful, just unbelievably tired. After all, I was doing what I needed to do while Jim was doing what he needed to do.

One day, the family from whom we had rented our house in Montgomery Village for two years suddenly came back to the States from Australia. We had to find another place to live starting that summer. And to add to the excitement of having to move again, Jim started talking about relocating all of us "overseas."

14

Walk Like an Egyptian

—Bangles

In the fall of 1994, when Benjamin was eight, Patrick was seven (as was I), and Kassidy was two, Jim started talking about the possibility of us moving overseas to one of two places: either to Bangkok, Thailand, or to Cairo, Egypt. He was working for a "global technologies group" at a consulting firm and all I really understood about that job was that he was away from home traveling most of the time. As far as I was concerned, "Bangkok" or "Cairo" could have just as well been Ohio or Pennsylvania, as I had no real concept of what "overseas" really meant. I can vaguely remember thinking that perhaps it was a kind of letter . . . "Over-C's" . . . like maybe it was a place that skipped "over" the letter *C* or something, although I had never seen an "Over-C" letter on *Sesame Street* . . .

I was not familiar with geography, and even though I watched Where in the World Is Carmen Sandiego? with Benjamin and Patrick, I didn't really understand that there were whole other continents and countries far away from where I lived with the kids in Montgomery Village. I did sometimes attempt to read the *Washington Post,* or at least look at the photographs, and when Jim was home, he sometimes watched the news on CNN. But again, the places that I read about and saw on TV were somehow in my mind *only* in the newspaper or on TV. It's hard to explain except to say I didn't connect what I read or saw with anything *real.* It wasn't until many years later that the paper or news on television actually held my attention for any length of time anyway.

The thought of moving again was not all that appealing to me initially. I was tired of the tedious process of packing up, and then unpacking, all our stuff. And then the worst part: learning where our belongings were in a new house. However, Jim kept telling the kids and me excitedly, "It will be an adventure!" That's a good thing, right? Jim came home from his long trips to Thailand bearing exotic gifts and talking about live elephants in the streets and huge extravagant palaces. He came home from Cairo with more extravagant gifts and stories of irritated camels and impressive pyramids. In addition to the "adventure" component, Jim convincingly explained that the family would get to be together because he wouldn't have to travel anymore. His job would be in just one place and he would get to come home at the end of each day. That was enough for me! Sign me up! I was tired of living as a single mom, on call 24/7. In addition, I was teaching at least fourteen aerobics and spin classes a week at four different gyms, trying to help out financially as much as possible. There never seemed to be quite enough money despite Jim's substantial salary as well as my own efforts. The thought that Jim might be able to help out with the kids—homework, the school morning routine, activities, meals, and bedtime—would certainly be a dream come true.

But it wasn't until March of 1996 that this move became a reality. In fact, it wasn't until early in January of that year that we even knew that we would be going to Cairo instead of Bangkok.

This move itself was extremely confusing because Jim kept saying that we (the kids and I) had to decide what we wanted to have with us in Cairo and what was going into "storage." I knew about Ziploc storage bags, but I had never heard the word *storage* used in the context of moving and I had never had to make these kinds of decisions before with any other move. Was this a money issue? Was "storage" a kind of store where our stuff would be sold to other people and we would never see it again? Or was our stuff going somewhere like the giant church yard sale? How could I possibly decide what possessions I wanted to keep? Jim said we would be in Cairo for up to three or four years. Exactly how long was that? I still had trouble keeping track of *daily* schedules. Concepts of years in the future were, and to a certain extent still are, beyond my comprehension. I had difficulty remembering decisions I made, and because of my unpredictability, Jim grew frustrated and then furious with me. Choices had to be made, and time was running short, but his anger just frightened me, and I became even more erratic, impulsive, and useless. In the end, Jim took over and determined what would go with us and what would stay. I was most likely none the wiser.

After a short visit with Jim's family, we flew out of Atlanta late one March evening with the thought that we could all sleep on this long flight to Frankfurt, Germany. For some unknown reason the times of these flights have always stuck in my head; nine hours and forty-four minutes to Frankfurt, and then four hours and forty-four minutes from Frankfurt to Cairo. Given the length of the flights, you would think that I would understand that Cairo, Egypt, was very far away from Maryland. And yet it never occurred to me exactly how far away we were going. We brought tons of baggage with us, between suitcases, carry-ons, and backpacks filled to overcapacity with toys, books, games, clothing, and snacks for each of us, because we had no idea how long it would take for our household goods to arrive and "get through customs." I could tell that "getting through customs" was a big deal because of the way Jim always said it, but I had no idea what it really meant, except that whatever it was, "getting through customs" might take a long time.

We were flying "business class" on Lufthansa airlines, which was incredibly exciting for the kids and me. There was lots of legroom, the seats were wide and comfortable, there were several choices of movies or TV shows to watch, or music to listen to, and the flight attendants were especially accommodating, doting on all my children a lot of the time. Benjamin, more than any of the three, took advantage of the flight attendants' good nature, talking with them incessantly. One attendant brought all my kids puppets of the Lufthansa mascot, which was some kind of bird.

Kassidy has never flown well, and the fact that we were in the "fancier" business class had no effect on her delicate constitution. As soon as we took off she looked at me pleadingly and said, "I don't like the smell of this airplane." Those words became *the* well-known "secret code" for, "I am going to throw up in about thirty seconds." And she did just that. She threw up all over herself, our seats, the floor, and me. This happened whenever we flew anywhere every single time we took off or landed for many years. Needless to say, I got much better at not only packing extra clothes and supplies for both Kassidy and myself, but at recognizing that particular "secret code" and immediately flying into action in an attempt to save our existing outfits, and those of anyone sitting or standing nearby.

We stayed overnight in a hotel attached to the Frankfurt airport. I don't remember doing this, but Jim assures me we did. I wonder how confused I was, and if I even slept. Early the next morning we boarded the flight that would take us to Cairo. All five of us were tired of traveling, and the kids were all hungry and especially whiny. As Jim slept, Benjamin and Patrick began beating on each other, and no sooner had I separated them than Patrick started teasing Kassidy, which started her whining. And this just continued . . . I can remember having a huge headache during most of this flight and thinking, I am *not* going to survive! I just want to go home! I guess I didn't really appreciate that I was, indeed, headed home.

~

My first impression of Egypt was that it smelled bad and was dirty. There seemed to be a not-so-thin layer of dirt or dust all over everything, even inside the airport. There was no toilet paper in the bathroom, and Kassidy was *not* happy about that, so I let her wipe her bottom with my sweatshirt. Patrick refused to even *enter* the bathroom. There were lots of imposing-looking men with gigantic guns. It was extremely hot, and this was just March. It seemed as though everyone was smoking cigarettes. There were enormous black biting flies that descended on us as soon as we walked outside. Wagdi, Jim's driver, was just about the nicest human being on the planet, *but* I thought I was going to die as we drove from the airport to our hotel in Heliopolis because there did not appear to be any traffic laws of any kind.

Everything was so very different; sights, smells, and sounds were like nothing I had ever experienced. It was as if all my senses were being accosted, forced to exist suddenly on some kind of "high-alert status," which made me very uncomfortable and anxious. But I had been taught that it was better for everyone if I could keep a positive exterior, no matter how exhausted or concerned I was, and so that's exactly what I did, even as we were all being hurled dangerously through the streets of Cairo in a small black Fiat with no seat belts. Is this what Jim had meant when he said that this move would be an "adventure"? I hoped not.

We arrived at Le Méridien, Heliopolis where we would live until we could get into a flat, and were immediately treated as if we were an important royal family. Everything was "Yes, Mister Jim, sir," "Right away, Mr. Jim sir." And my kids became almost instantly the darlings of Le Méridien. No sooner had we arrived than Kassidy, with her blond curls and huge blue eyes, thoroughly won over Mustafa, the enormous friendly doorman. And both boys, no matter what mayhem they brought to this fancy five-star hotel (and trust me, they brought plenty!) could do no wrong as far as the staff was concerned, even though we were there for four months. I can remember both boys being ushered back to our room on several occasions by members of the hotel staff. If I sent them to fill the ice bucket, they would end up playing in the elevators, having a great time riding it up and down. Sometimes they would just slip out of our suite and race through the long straight hallways. Or they would find their way down to the enormous fancy lobby, where there was a bakery, some shops and restaurants, and crowds of fascinating people to watch. Did I even realize when they were gone for long stretches of time? And what about the serious trouble they could have—and may well have—gotten themselves into? What about the danger? They could have easily been kidnapped or severely injured as they ran around unattended.

We had two large connected hotel rooms for the five of us and we were given a small refrigerator. Jim would get up and go to work fairly early each morning, and he and Wagdi repeatedly told me never to leave the hotel unless they were with me. I kept the shades drawn, which made the rooms very dark, and the kids and I would sleep until almost noon. When I think back on it now, the four of us just stayed more or less on eastern standard time rather than shifting to local Cairo time, because . . . well . . . we could. When we eventually did wake up, the kids would watch TV while I made breakfast. I can remember making Tang with bottled water, washing apples and grapes with bottled water, eating cereal out of the box with no milk—because the milk was gross—as well as making tuna fish and peanut butter and jelly sandwiches. The hotel had Star TV, which was a channel with an abundance of the old American TV shows like *Brady Bunch, Partridge Family, Remington Steele, Lost in Space, H.R. Pufnstuf, The Monkees, Black Beauty,* and *MacGyver*. Every single one of these TV shows was just as new and fresh to me as they were to the kids. I have *never* watched so much television, and allowed my children to watch so much, as we did during those first months in Cairo.

After a few hours of TV and food, we would all throw on our bathing suits, slap on sunscreen, and head out to camp at the pool. Benjamin taught Kassidy to swim without her floaties that spring before she turned four. I was afraid of the water, so I certainly couldn't teach her, but I was always full of encouragement. We had toy Gumby and Pokey figures with us that would sink, and Kassidy would scramble down the stairs of the pool and swim out to "save them." Patrick changed his name to "Max" soon after arriving in Cairo because "Patrick" sounded similar to an Arabic word meaning "shoes" or "sneakers." He stayed Max the entire time we lived in Cairo. On the pool deck, we would order strawberry smoothies almost daily. And we played the card games War and Pocahontas and the board game *Rummikub Junior.* I also attempted to read the Beatrix Potter books aloud, all twenty-four of them, repeatedly, as they were initially the only "picture books" we had with us.

As the afternoon would down, we would head in for a "parade of showers," get dressed for dinner, and then sit and watch some more TV while we waited for Jim to arrive. When he was late we would all get hungry and snack on the Egyptian version of Cheez-Its, plus fruit and cereal. As soon as Jim returned to our suite, we headed out to have dinner. We would walk past President Mubarak's palace compound and end up at either Chili's, Planet Hollywood, or McDonald's. If we had Wagdi to drive us, we often had him drive us all the way to Maadi to eat at Arby's or Pizza Hut. Then it was back to the hotel for more TV and bedtime. We had pretty much this same routine day in and day out for more than four months. There were slight variations during those weekends when Jim did not have to work, which, regrettably, wasn't too often. But on those days, Jim would have Wagdi drive us to the Tiba Mall, or the Alpha Market, or to Maadi, where we would begin the search for a flat to live in once our stuff "made it through customs."

During the last days of May, Jim had to travel to Alexandria

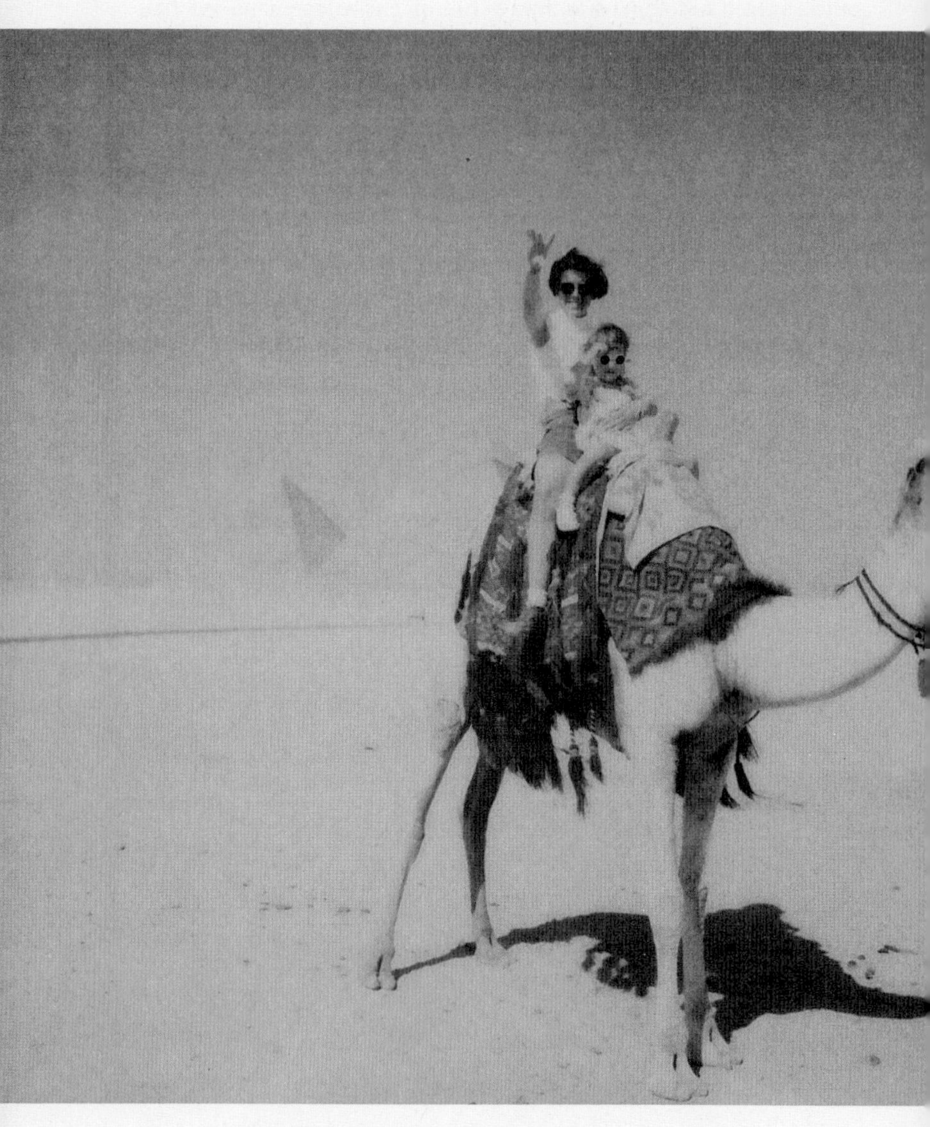

Kassidy and me on a camel our first spring in Cairo

for work. And because I was going absolutely stir-crazy living in the hotel by myself with my kids, the four of us went along with him for a change of scenery. We took the train, and during the trip, Benjamin looked out his window and noticed lots of people outside, quite literally, living in boxes in the desert between Cairo and Alexandria. But instead of thinking, Oh, those poor people living in boxes in the desert, he said with genuine admiration, "Wow Mom! Look! They really know how to recycle in this country!"

Jim says we celebrated Benjamin's tenth birthday together that weekend on June 1, 1996, in a beautiful hotel overlooking the Mediterranean Sea. I wish I could remember more about it. I wish I could remember what I thought when I saw the Mediterranean Sea. Unfortunately, the whole trip was probably just more perplexing to me because other than Benjamin's birthday festivities, it was basically trading one unfamiliar hotel for another. Jim probably told us we shouldn't go anywhere, and he most likely worked the whole time.

Kassidy celebrated her fourth birthday back at Le Méridien Hotel in Heliopolis the following month, on July 13. The chef in the fancy French bakery baked her an enormous, and voguely alarming, Mickey Mouse cake and delivered it to our room. Wagdi bought her a stuffed bear that Kassidy named "Tiba" after the Tiba Mall in Nasr City, halfway between Heliopolis and Maadi. Kassidy probably asked to go to the Tiba Mall that evening. On the roof, or somewhere near the roof, of the mall there were all these kiddie rides, like you might see at an amusement park, but an old amusement park from the 1950s or 1960s. Lots of bright pink and turquoise and exaggerated animal characters. There were also really old bumper cars that smelled weird. I always got really nervous when the kids wanted to ride those rides, because to me they didn't look at all safe. Isn't that strange? I didn't get one bit concerned about them running around in the hotel for hours at a time, where they could have been kidnapped or fallen down an elevator shaft, but I was afraid that they would get hurt on these rides at Tiba Mall. How odd is that?

~

Finally, in August, after more than four months in Egypt, we were freed from the confines of hotel life. We moved into an enormous flat in Maadi before our stuff actually arrived because we wanted to get the boys acclimated to that area and have them meet some other kids before starting school in September. Maadi is the area in Cairo where most expats lived, mainly because Cairo American College (CAC), the American School for grades K through 12, is located there. Unfortunately, most families were away traveling in August, so there were not too many people around for the boys to meet and play with. But the four of us did spend a lot of time exploring and familiarizing ourselves with the grounds of the school—the playgrounds, the soccer fields, and the Olympic-size swimming pool and diving well. Because there was nothing to really do in the flat until our stuff arrived, we also spent lots of time outside investigating the community of Maadi and discovering things like a grocery store, Gomma Digla; the post office, and Road 9, a stretch of shops and restaurants. There were also gorgeous softball fields in Maadi, where I eventually played first base and became one of the league's top home-run hitters for the ex-pat team the Jewels of the Nile and the all-star team the Cairo Cruisers.

I had never had a hard time finding work in health clubs before, and I thought that there would be dozens of gyms needing instructors in Cairo just like in Maryland. But there weren't. I don't exactly know how I found out about Samia Aluba's Creative Dance and Fitness. Maybe it was something that Wagdi told us about, or maybe the real estate people who were showing us available flats in Maadi, or someone at Cairo American College when we registered the boys for school, I honestly don't know. I also don't recall any kind of interview or audition process with Samia, although I'm sure there was some sort of official hiring procedure. I do think that I started teaching classes there in the evenings before we moved to Maadi, while we were still living in the hotel. Jim recalls that Wagdi would drive all five of us to Maadi, and I would teach a class while he and Wagdi took the kids to play or swim at Cairo American College.

Creative Dance and Fitness was a very different sort of club from the ones I knew. A lot of the equipment was unfamiliar, people wore unusual workout attire and shoes, some of the music was strange to my ears, and to me the safety, education, and training techniques were different. It was a very small club overall, but the aerobics studio was quite large and airy, with huge windows along the whole back wall. I loved teaching classes in that room! And I loved working for Samia. She was the most amazing person, well educated and well spoken, beautiful, smart, kind, and in fabulous shape. Because her studio was in Maadi, everyone spoke English, but there were some distinctive customs that I had to learn. For example, we instructors were *never* allowed to set up our own steps; there were paid "boys" for that. And the same went for other equipment as well, whether it was mats, weights, or straps. Some of my aerobics music was deemed "inappropriate," and Samia very gently explained to me that she did not want members to be offended by provocative lyrics. To be honest, I had never really listened to many of the lyrics on my pre-made aerobics tapes. I mostly only paid attention to the speed and the beat of the music. The same went for what I wore. There were a few women who regularly took classes in long loose garments. Their arms, legs, and bodies were, for the most part, fully covered. Samia warmly (but firmly) suggested to me early on that I wear T-shirts over my tiny jog bras when I taught. Obviously not everyone who belonged to this studio was Egyptian or even Muslim. And certainly not all of the Egyptian Muslims who showed up to take my classes would have been offended by my music or dress, but Samia kept a certain standard, and she was respected for that.

I had not been teaching at Samia's club for too long when I approached her and asked if I might be able to put together some kind of training program for the other instructors. (After all, I had been teaching for all of five or six years, so I was *obviously* an expert.) After learning to teach aerobics in the litigious society that was suburban Washington, D.C., I was hyperaware of the many "contraindicated aspects of exercise" that should *never be done* in any group setting. When I noticed many movements were being done improperly in other classes in Samia's studio, I think it drove me a little bit crazy. I had been always told in no uncertain terms that there were "proper" and "correct" and "acceptable" ways of warming up, stretching, and teaching various movements in order to avoid injury. It had been all but beaten into me while teaching at previous gyms that anything that deviated from the correct ways was not only wrong but also downright harmful. And let's not forget that I was (am) a *total* rule follower, with a definite *right* way and a definite *wrong* way to do stuff.

Surprisingly, Samia agreed to let me set up a little training program for her instructors. She also suggested that any other members who were interested in learning more specifically about safety, and more generally about other teaching techniques, were welcome to attend. Little did I realize then the rabbit hole I was headed down. Not all of Samia's instructors were on board with this in-house training of mine, but enough people were that I considered it a success. I ended up using my copy of the ACE (American Council on Exercise) manual to teach from because there were lots of pictures that I understood. This way I thought I could easily explain to people the "whys" and "why not's" of group exercise. Several attendees of this program approached me and Samia afterward, and asked about the manual I had used and where they could buy their own copies. I explained about ACE, and that the books were only sent to people who were interested in becoming ACE-certified aerobics instructors.

Before I knew what had happened, Samia had ordered a dozen ACE Aerobics Instructor Manuals, and put me in charge of teaching a course to interested members and instructors who wanted to become ACE-certified instructors! I had no clue what I had gotten myself into, but fortunately for me, everyone who decided to sign up and take this class, as well as Samia herself, was eager, enthusiastic, and motivated, in addition to being extremely patient with me. Little by little, week after week, my confidence increased. I did have a lot of practical experience teaching, and I became better at figuring stuff out, even if I couldn't always read and understand the exact technicalities of everything written in the manual. Samia helped me set up a CPR (cardiopulmonary resuscitation) course to be taught at Cairo American College specifically for these twelve people, as well as an ACE (American Council on Exercise) examination team, which included proctors, to come to Cairo in order to administer the ACE Aerobics Instructor Exam. In the end, I think (but am not 100 percent sure) that all twelve that took the exam, passed. And many of the people that started out just as interested participants began teaching at Creative Dance and Fitness soon after successfully completing the class and the exam.

When I left Cairo, Samia threw a big party. She and other members contributed to a gift fund, and bought me a twenty-four-karat-gold cartouche with my name, Susan, in hieroglyphics. I haven't taken it off since it was given to me back in the spring of 1997.

~

School started up in September. Benjamin and Patrick attended Cario American College and I enrolled Kassidy in a Montessori preschool program close by. This was the first time I had all three kids in school. And even though Kassidy was just gone for a few hours in the mornings, it gave me time to teach aerobics at Creative Dance and Fitness without experiencing the guilt that I always felt when I had to put the kids in the nursery in order to work. I volunteered in both of the boys' classrooms once or twice a week, reading aloud, organizing graded papers, or helping with bulletin boards.

The school week in Egypt went from Sunday to Thursday, with Friday and Saturday as the weekend. The majority of expats spent most of every Friday at the softball fields because almost everywhere else was closed, as Friday is the holy day for Muslims. I cannot remember playing softball before going to Egypt, and I have no recollection of being taught how to play, but by far the happiest memories I have of all our time in Cairo are those that occurred on those softball fields. God, it was a blast! Herb was our coach, 100 percent Texan, through and through. Alison, his Aussie girlfriend, played shortstop, and her best friend, Ruthie, also an

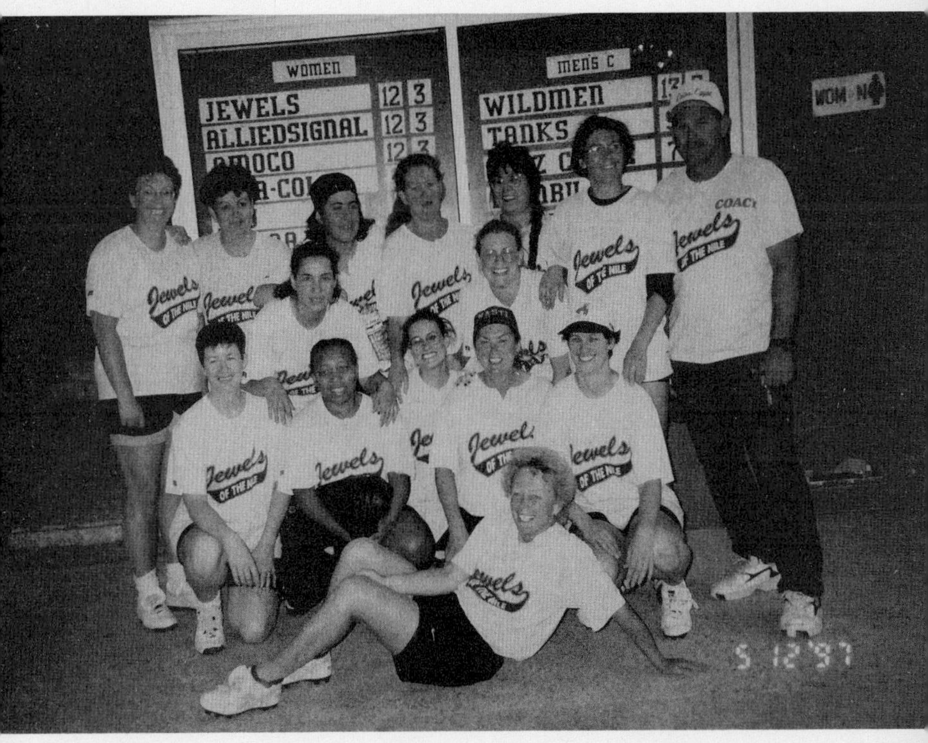

The Jewels of the Nile. I am standing next to Herb, our coach, and my friend Heather Corkin is in the first row of kneelers all the way on the left side. The Jewels are ranked first on the standings board behind us.

Aussie with flaming-red hair, was either our pitcher or catcher depending on the lineup. My good friend Heather Corkin, a "Kiwi" from New Zealand, played second base or in the outfield, as did my friend Valerie, another American. Being a lefty, with long legs, I played first base exclusively. I caught nearly anything and everything that was ever thrown to or at me, while often having to stretch in order to keep my foot on the bag. I was also a particularly fast runner, nicknamed "Cheetah" by my teammates, and I was a strong power hitter, especially when Herb let me use his double wall bat. However, I never quite got a handle on the throwing part, and I pretty much always sucked whenever I had to throw the ball.

So much of life doesn't always turn out the way you think it will. I always believed and trusted Jim, and I hoped that when we moved to Egypt, we would be able to live as a family of five, with two parents working equally as parents to *our* three children. Unfortunately, Jim was just as much of a workaholic as he had always been. And even though he didn't have to travel, per se, he still worked absurdly long hours, as well as most weekends, so the kids and I still rarely saw him. I was just as exhausted a single parent in Cairo as I had ever been living in Maryland. Jim did hire Emiline, a Filipina maid, to help with the cleaning, as it was nearly impossible to keep up with the dust and dirt that seemed to relentlessly seep through the tiny cracks in the windows and doors to cover any and every surface. But the children, with their schoolwork, activities, meals, bedtimes, not to mention each of their individual adjustments to a new home, school, classmates, teachers, culture, food. . . . all of that fell to me.

I wasn't adjusting too well to the substantial changes in my life, either. I enjoyed teaching aerobics, and I loved playing softball, but there was a lot that was getting to me. As a relatively selfish American, coming from a fairly upper middle-class suburb, I was used to having electricity, water, and phone service most if not all the time. In Cairo, we would have one of those things, occasionally two, but never all three. The kids and I were stranded in the tiny elevator once early on when the power went out; nobody (myself included) wanted to ride that elevator ever again. That was five flights up and five flights down with a four-year-old whenever I wanted to go anywhere. The flies and mosquitoes were persistent in and outside the flat. I got tired of feeling dirty and dusty all of the time. I was both dependent on, and limited by, my bike and the Burley trailer to go anywhere or do anything. If I needed to go grocery shopping, for example, and I had Kassidy with me, I was limited to buying only what I could fit into the trailer alongside her. There was just so much change for me to try to understand all at once.

Poverty surrounded us. There were tiny, very young children driving donkey carts full of garbage or, worse, canisters of kerosene. Once there was a woman screaming for seemingly the entire night in the hovel next door to our building, and the next day when I walked the boys to the bus stop for school, there were the bloody remains of a dead baby lying alongside the road. Most days, Patrick insisted I walk them to the bus. He was afraid to walk by a scruffy territorial rooster that would chase anyone who went near it. The blind man with no teeth whom we always passed on our bikes getting to Road 9; the dozens of dirty, naked children that lived and played in the garbage at the dump got to me. And all the stray animals got to me too. There were literally hundreds of stray dogs and cats everywhere we went. We "adopted" two cats, Amber and Alexander, but I could have adopted two thousand cats and dogs and it still would not have made any difference. I missed talking to my family, especially my parents. Phone calls to the States were extremely expensive and even though we had a computer, we didn't have the ability to send e-mail from our flat. Everything was just so unfamiliar.

Eventually the challenges of trying to navigate this puzzling place without the support of family and friends drove me to the breaking point. I don't think it was anything more than Jim working yet another weekend, but I had had enough. I don't know if I was tired, or if I was confused, or if I was just plain lonely, but when Wagdi showed up to drive Jim to work, I started shouting, crying, pleading, and threatening. I have no idea where the kids were, but if I were to speculate, I would guess that Benjamin had gathered his brother and sister into their room, closed the door, and played games or read books with them, as was his habit when Jim and I fought. I also don't know how it all ended. Again, I would guess that Jim left me there and went to work anyway, absolutely furious with me for embarrassing him in front of Wagdi as well as messing with him when he was just trying to "do my job!" Later, I imagine everything was just "normal" and nobody would ever speak of the incident again. Jim says by the time he returned from work, I had forgotten the whole thing. In fact, this was one of those stories that I heard for the first time when Jim was recounting his own memories from Cairo for this book. He says now he never knew or really understood how hard it was for me living there. To him, that particular enormous emotional explosion of mine came out of nowhere. He wasn't worried, because he recalls that I had a habit of being overly dramatic, and he had to get to work. What he considered my tendency to be overly dramatic was in fact genuine distress and considerable anxiety that he just never noticed as such.

At Thanksgiving, we traveled to Luxor with another American

family with whom we had become close. They were initially my "go to" people when I had questions about where I could get peanut butter, where I could find books written in English and school supplies for the boys, and who to call when there were rats as big as large cats in our flat. They invited us to go along with them to Crocodile Island, a resort area in the southern part of Egypt near Luxor. My most vivid memory of that resort was Kassidy getting bitten by a goat, and me wondering and worrying for the rest of the time if goats carried rabies. Jim says we played a lot of tennis, and the kids played in an enormous swimming pool. We apparently had a Thanksgiving-like dinner in the main dining room that reminded Benjamin of camp because there were long wooden tables.

At Christmastime, we traveled to my brother's family's house outside of Dayton, Ohio, and later we met up with my sister and her family as well as Jim's parents in Williamsburg, Virginia. I don't honestly remember anything at all about that Christmas, until the very end. We were back in the Holiday Inn in Gaithersburg, and Jim was on the phone with Jack, his big boss at his D.C. office. I was trying to keep the kids as quiet as I could while getting them ready for bed. When Jim got off the phone, he announced that he was going to be recalled to the States. Apparently, working twenty-+ hours a day seven days a week wasn't good enough for Jim's boss, who essentially said to Jim during this phone call, "If we had wanted you to have a wife and family, we would have issued you one."

I could see the strain and feel Jim's panic, so I kept very quiet. I had learned a long time ago that I was utterly useless in times of crisis, even though at this moment I had so many questions I wanted to ask. Were we going to fly all the way back to Cairo now, just to fly back in another month? Where would we return to anyway? We had no house, no car, nothing we could come back to, as far as I could see. Where would the kids go to school? What about the great school where they were already enrolled in Maadi? Benjamin had *never* had such a great year as he was having at Cairo American College. What about my job and softball team in Cairo? I didn't understand how all of this would fit together, or how any of it would work. So I just swallowed hard and went into supportive and silent wife mode.

~

As it turned out, we all flew back to Cairo without any real plans. Back in Maadi, we continued to make it up as we went along. Jim had to go back to Maryland. That much was made clear. Movers came within the month and packed us up. (Hadn't we just done this?) Jim went back to Montgomery County and lived in the basement of our ex-next door neighbors, Moira and Jerry LaVeck. Heather Corkin, from my softball team, and her husband, Alan, were generous enough to let the kids and me move into their flat with them and their three kids until the end of the school year in June. Jim figured he would be able to find us a place to live by then, and we could all move back to Maryland as soon as the boys finished school. Kassidy would be able to finish her year of preschool, and I would be able to tell Samia that I would be leaving come June, instead of just disappearing with no notice. It sounded like a doable plan. But once again, I was left by myself with responsibility for the kids. Or maybe from their perspective, they were left by themselves with responsibility for their mom.

The Corkin family lived directly across the street from Cairo American College, so it was more convenient for the kids to get to and from school. Their flat was also much closer to Kassidy's preschool, and my job at Creative Dance and Fitness. Nevertheless it certainly was not the most ideal situation for anyone, with three adults and six children from ages four to eleven, all living in a single flat. We all tried to keep an upbeat attitude and I'll be the first to admit that I certainly didn't always succeed. Especially toward the end. Heather and I did spend a lot of our time laughing, but morning routines, homework, meals, and bedtime were sometimes absolute chaos. I had horrific headaches most of the time, and I often felt lost and confused, forgetting why we were there. The kids and I all slept in one bed during those months. On one hand I don't know how much sleep I ever got, and yet, on the other, I was completely thankful that we had a place to stay.

At one point early in the spring while we were living with the Corkins, a massive sandstorm blew through Maadi. Heather and I had all six kids with us at the softball fields, where we were finishing up a practice with the Jewels. I remember feeling a sudden shift in the air and detecting an unpleasant smell. Herb swore, and he said that everyone needed to get indoors immediately. Heather and I lived pretty close by, so we gathered all the kids at once and rode our bikes back to the flat as quickly as we could. We didn't quite make it before there was a wall of wind and dirt upon us. The storm probably didn't last any more than half an hour—maybe less—but it was one of the most terrifying things I had ever experienced. The wind was howling, and sand and stones were being pelted against the windows of the flat. None of us could hear a thing except the roar of the storm, and we couldn't see our own hands in front of our faces. By the end, all the windows in the front room of the flat were blown in. I can remember Heather and me just looking at each other and laughing. What else was there to do? The flat was an absolute disaster. There were literally inches of dirt and dust on the floor, covering every surface, and all eight of us were completely and utterly filthy. There was broken glass everywhere and both Heather's daughter Cara and Kassidy were running around with bare feet because in our rush to leave the softball fields, we had left their sandals.

In February or early March, Heather and Alan decided to take some time to go away together. I had recently been chosen to play first base for the women's all-star softball team, the Cairo Cruisers, who would be traveling to the United Arab Emirates to play in a big tournament during the first week of April. Heather and Alan agreed to look after Benjamin, Patrick, and Kassidy while I was away if I agreed to care for Tracy, Alex, and Cara while they went away for their holiday. It seemed to me like a fair trade. I knew that my boys were much more difficult to handle than the Corkin kids, and if this deal meant that I could travel unencumbered to the UAE just by taking care of all six for a few days, I thought, Great! It's a deal!

The funny thing is, I can remember sitting down with Heather and Alan and hammering out all the details of, and making preparations for, our kid trade arrangement, but I have next to no recollections of staying by myself with all six children. I don't know if this means that everything went beautifully, with no problems whatsoever, or if I just think it did because I don't recall anything especially horrible. I can't imagine what it must have been like getting everyone ready for school each morning. Tracy, Alex, Benjamin, and Patrick all could easily walk across the street to CAC. But what about getting everyone up, dressed, fed, and out the door? Cara and Kassidy attended different preschools, so each morning they must have ridden in the bike trailer together, and I must have dropped them each off separately. CAC didn't have a cafeteria, so I must have made six different lunches each morning. I wonder if anyone did any homework that week. Or took baths. Bedtime must have been chaotic as well. As I write this, I do have a vague recollection of Cara howling as I tried to brush out her hair. I think Tracy was most likely my biggest source of help and support that week.

Jim flew to Cairo that Spring, and came with me to the softball tournament in UAE. All the travel arrangements, like flights, a bus and driver, hotel rooms, and I think even meals, were organized for us ahead of time. From a post-9/11 perspective, I can't imagine all of us just waltzing onto the airplane with our gear bags, complete with mitts and *softball bats,* but I'm certain that is what we all did, and we probably didn't think anything of it.

I have never been back, but I do remember that in 1997 the United Arab Emirates was the most sparkling and gorgeous country that I had ever visited. The beaches of Abu Dhabi along the Persian Gulf were absolutely pristine. Everything in Dubai, from the buildings, to the shopping areas, to the roads, to cars, and even the people themselves seemed to be clean, shiny, and brand-new. The softball fields where we played were spectacular, with actual grass in the outfields, and the stands for spectators were comfortable and shaded, a far cry from those in Maadi. I am thinking that the Cairo Cruisers as a team didn't do very well during this particular tournament, but we all had a great time together as a team, getting to play against, as well as watch, some really impressive teams. Jim and I enjoyed ourselves thoroughly as well. This was the first time since Kathy and Randy's wedding five years before that we had gone away together. Just the two of us, with no kids.

~

Back in Cairo, the kids and I were keeping track of the days on a calendar in our bathroom at the Corkins'. Each evening, one of us would cross off another day as we counted down to the end of the school year when we would be heading back to Montgomery County. The Corkin family was generous with their computer, and the four of us together e-mailed back and forth almost every day with Jim and also with my parents. Jim sent us e-mails about the neighborhoods and houses he was looking at. Kassidy kept asking if we could get a dog when we got back. Patrick wanted to know if he could have his own room. Benjamin was lobbying hard for a Game Boy system for the long plane ride home. I think somewhere deep down, I *knew* that I was going to have to get the kids and myself back to Maryland from Cairo without Jim come June. But because I had no concept of how I would actually *do* that, I never came up with any kind of a plan. Here again was another example of the whole concept of time and planning that I sucked at so badly! It's not like we had a lot of stuff to pack up. The moving van in January had taken everything except the clothes we wore, some books, and a few personal items. I am not sure what happened to our bikes and the trailer, but other than these, everything we had fit into our suitcases.

I have to say that I am unbelievably grateful to everyone in the Corkin family—Heather, Alan, Tracy, Alex, and Cara—for their hospitality and generosity during those six months. But all nine of us living under one roof unfortunately *did* get old. With the exception of Cara and Kassidy, who rarely argued and always played so well together, the kids began to irritate each other, and Heather and I began getting on each other's nerves as well. I am sorry now for the way that I acted toward her at the end of our stay in Cairo. Heather and I were terrific friends, essentially from our first meeting. We both loved our kids more than anything. Neither of us was especially stuffy and proper in the way we lived and raised our children. We enjoyed a lot of the same music. We both had fun playing softball and working out together. And we laughed most all of the time we were together. However, at the end, the laughter and fun were totally gone, and one day after school let out for the summer, I packed up the kids and myself and we left for Heliopolis and Le Méridien. Being back in that hotel felt like coming home somehow. We stayed there for a few days, and then flew back to Maryland. I never actually said good-bye and thank you to Heather and her family. That particular fact has bothered me for years.

15

Shiny Happy People

—R.E.M.

We arrived at Dulles Airport, exhausted, after traveling for more than thirty-six hours. Kassidy, a shaky traveler at the best of times, had thrown up all over herself and on me repeatedly, but because I had invested in Game Boys for both boys, everyone was, for the most part, intact. It was great to be back in the States after being in Cairo with the kids for what felt like a decade when in reality it was just under two years. The things we take for granted in this country: toilet paper, Kleenex tissues, Jif peanut butter, electricity, clean drinking water directly from the tap, traffic laws, driving, milk, Goldfish crackers, hamburger, ham, and Target! . . . I enjoyed many things in Egypt and I made some great friends while living there, but it was still good to be back.

Not that everything was instantly familiar. Jim bought us a house in Montgomery County, but it was nowhere near where we had lived before in Montgomery Village. Jim had done extensive research on the schools in the different areas of the county and had determined that the Wootton High School cluster zip codes had the highest SAT score of any that we could afford. It was a good choice of home for our family in a terrific neighborhood.

Jim took us right from the airport to see our new house. I remember feeling so exhausted and filthy that all I wanted was a shower and a bed, but Jim was too excited for us to see our home and couldn't wait any longer. The kids were excited, too, so off we went. It was a split-level with four bedrooms, three full baths, a beautiful newly remodeled kitchen and deck, a den, dining room, family room, living room, laundry room, and a large walk-out basement. There was a surprising amount of living space in that house, but not much closet or storage space. It had a one-car garage, and a large fenced backyard with a swing set. There was a forest of dense bamboo along two sides of the backyard that served as a barrier between our backyard and Darnestown Road. Because of this bamboo, we early on began referring to our new home as "Bamboo Corners." I sat down on the hardwood floor in the family room and stared at the beautiful kitchen and, without even exploring any of the rest of the house I said "Honey, you did great! This is perfect!" As I sat on that floor, it was easy to imagine that this was the home where my life would *finally* start to make more sense.

Benjamin, Patrick, and Kassidy were all wild! A huge empty house that they could explore, dashing from one room to another, was exactly what they needed to release their pent up energy. They all picked out their bedrooms first. Patrick's was light green with fish stenciled on the walls, and Kassidy's was Pepto-Bismol pink

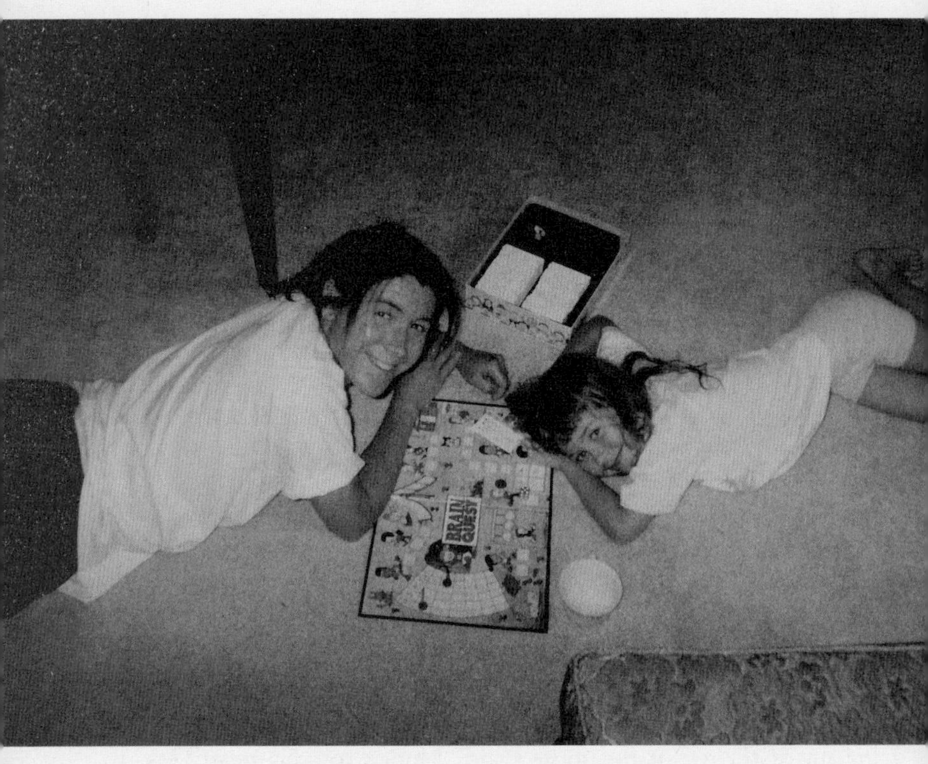

Kassidy and I played games together all the time. She usually kicked my ass whenever we played Brain Quest.

with a *beautiful* ballet shoe border. She loved it! Benjamin and Patrick decided they were going to share the fish room initially so we could keep one room as a guest room, but that only lasted a few months and the guest room became Benjamin's room.

All three kids found Super Balls somewhere and started throwing and bouncing them all over the family room, where I was sitting half asleep. Okay! Time to go. But first Kassidy had to know, "Where is my dog?" We had promised the kids that we would get a dog when we got back to Maryland. We were back in Maryland now, so where was the dog? Five-year-old logic at its very best.

We took a short walk up to see the Westleigh Community pool and tennis courts before piling back into the car. Jim had flown to his parents' house in Georgia before we arrived home from Egypt and had been given their old car. An extremely generous gift. And it wasn't long before we were also the proud owners of a purple Plymouth Grand Voyager named Jewel, after my softball team in Cairo, the Jewels of the Nile.

I was not yet going to get my shower and bed because Jim wanted to show the kiddos where they would be going to school. Kassidy was tremendously excited to be starting kindergarten come fall, Patrick would possibly be repeating fourth grade, and Benjamin would be heading to middle school. Jim drove by Dufief Elementary School first because it was close. We got lost looking for Robert Frost Middle School, so we gave up and went to the Woodfin Suites, where we stayed until closing on our house the following weekend.

For the first time *ever,* Jim took time off work and helped out with this move into "Bamboo Corners." And things went relatively smoothly, although there were so many boxes piled everywhere. We had boxes and furniture that came directly to us from Egypt, as well as boxes that we had placed in storage before moving to Cairo. Opening up the boxes that had been in storage was like discovering an entirely different household. Everything was brand-new to me. I started to panic. This wasn't our stuff. I had absolutely no recollection of those particular plates, glasses, books, towels, sheets, dresses, boots, coats, or toys. It was a strange sensation, because it felt as though we had gotten somebody else's stuff delivered to our house. Wouldn't those people wonder where their stuff was? Jim, with his usual impatience, told me to just stop freaking out, unpack it, and put it away.

Early in the fall of 1997, we fulfilled a promise to Kassidy and adopted two gorgeous Lab puppies from the organization Lab Rescue: Linus, a roly-poly chocolate Lab boy, and Lucy, a beautiful tiny black Lab girl. Amber and Alexander, the two cats that we brought back from Cairo, were utterly dismayed when Lucy and Linus first arrived, but eventually everyone got along just fine. Guess who ended up taking care of both the dogs and both cats most of the time? Jim would walk the dogs with me on nights he was in town, and the kids, especially Kassidy, would walk with me, too, but pretty much everything else fell to me. I was on feeding duty, poop duty, bath and brush duty, daytime walk duty, and vacuuming-pet-hair duty. But I loved those dogs, and their unconditional dog love got me through some tough times. (I loved the cats, too, but their love was always a bit more contingency based.)

But my life back in Montgomery County, was often chaotic, especially during the school year. Because Benjamin and Patrick had both been diagnosed with ADHD and other learning difficulties, they were required to have Individualized Education Programs (IEPs). What this meant in the Montgomery County Public School was a lot of meetings to discuss appropriate levels

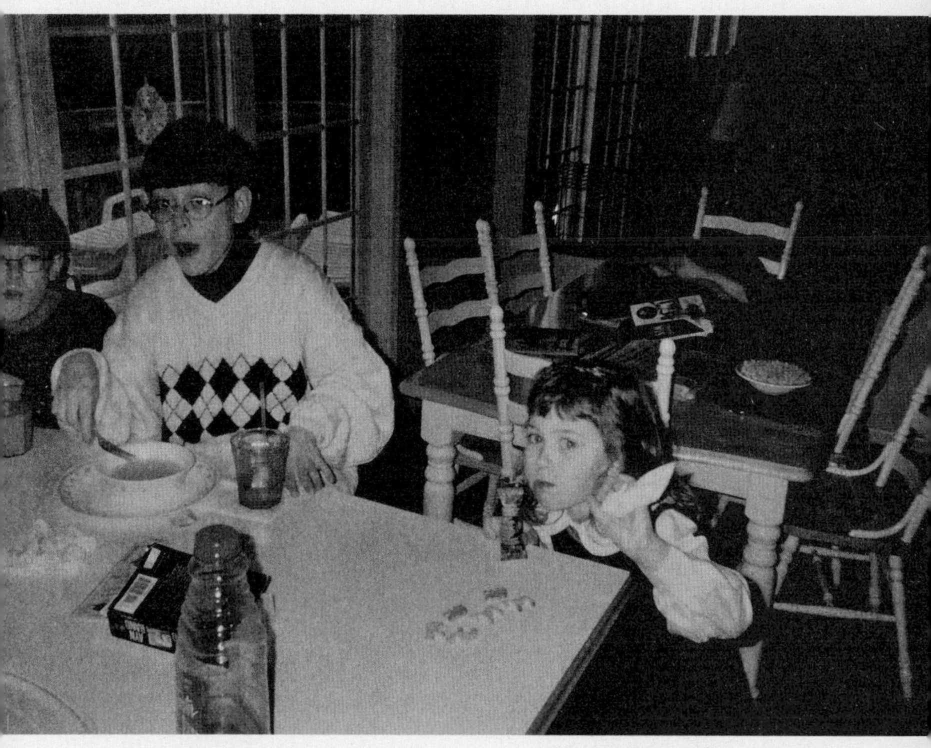

Dinners at our house were often unusual. Here Patrick is eating toast, Benjamin is eating soup with a fork because he only liked the noodles, and Kassidy is eating animal crackers. On the table behind the kids sits my bowl of Cap'n Crunch.

of disability support services, lots of signed papers and documentation about the different kinds of classroom accommodations that might be suitable, then more meetings with classroom teachers who didn't believe in making *any* classroom accommodations for students, many times having to change schedules in order to get teachers who might follow the IEP, and finally lots of extra doctor's appointments for appropriate-dosage medication checkups.

For the first couple of years after we got back from overseas, Jim worked for a small system integration company, and he didn't have to travel too much. He went with me to many of those IEP meetings for the boys at their schools if they were scheduled early enough in the morning or late enough in the afternoon. That is, he went with me until he shouted at Benjamin's administrator and made Benjamin's special educator, Wendy Salzman, cry. Then he didn't go to any more meetings for a few years. In fact, on the letters that came ever after, there was always a handwritten question at the bottom: "Will Mr. Meck be joining us for this meeting?"

During the fall of 1998, Jim was diagnosed with Lyme disease and was on IV antibiotics for six months. An IV pole lived in our bedroom, and every evening when Jim returned home from work, he would lie in bed and medicine would drip into his arm through an inserted catheter. A nurse came once a week to check his catheter for possible infection and to bring him his week's supply of antibiotics bags. Soon after that he lost his job. His next company was Protegrity, a commercial security software company, and his job there had him back on the road most of the time. With this company, Jim was responsible for North American pre-engineering sales.

I was teaching a bunch of each week at two different gyms, and all three kids were always involved in lots of activities over the years. I let them try whatever it was they were interested in for any given year. The only rule was that they had to finish out the season or semester of whatever they started; they weren't allowed to quit in the middle. Both Benjamin and Kassidy ultimately found their talents were best suited for musical theater. With musical theater came voice lessons, dance classes, and an endless string of auditions, shows, and recitals. But before that, Benjamin had tried violin, soccer, baseball, gymnastics, karate, rock climbing, math club, swim team, and improv team. Kassidy had taken dance classes from the time she was three before going to Egypt, but she had also tried soccer, horseback riding, gymnastics, swim team, track and field, and diving. They also both sang in choir and played handbells at church, and took piano lessons for several years. Patrick ended up as a nationally ranked platform diver in college. But before that he sang and rang in choirs for a couple of years, played soccer, took gymnastics classes, art lessons, photography classes, and had been part of chess club, cross-country, and the mass-driver club. My point is I lived in my car for more than ten years.

But, you may say, a lot of moms do that. In fact, most moms these days schlep their kids to and from dozens of activities. The difference with me was there was no rhyme or reason to the kids' schedules. For example, if Kassidy came and told me she wanted to take horseback riding lessons, I would say, "Sure," and just sign her up for horseback riding lessons on Thursdays from 4:00–5:30, not necessarily making a connection that Patrick's gymnastics class was already on Thursdays from four to five-fifteen in a totally different part of town. Or that Benjamin's jazz class was also on Thursdays from six to seven-thirty in yet another part of town. All this during rush hour in Montgomery County. Because I wasn't able, for whatever reason, to make connections between one thing and another, our lives were a hectic, jumbled, disorganized mess most of the time. I often forgot to pick up one kid or drop off another at the proper time. Other mothers did not like to carpool with me.

Jim recently has begun referring to this behavior of mine as "Now. Not now." My brain, since the injury, is happiest in the present, and for some unknown reason it is very unhappy in both the past and the future. If I am forced to think of something that happened last month, I have to literally walk myself backward through time in my head one small step at a time, attaching myself to other things that have happened. The future is much harder for me to walk forward into because there are no events that have yet happened for me to attach to. If something is happening in my life right now at this very instant—for example, Benjamin is making a fire in the fireplace—I can make sense of that thing and know that it is happening right now. Benjamin is making a fire in the fireplace. If next week I have to look back and remember that Benjamin made a fire in the fireplace, I have to think of lots of other "present" moments that happened throughout the week in order to walk back until I come to the specific "present moment" when Benjamin was making a fire in the fireplace. None of this happens automatically. I actually have to think about it for a long time. If I get the least little bit lost in my mind, if I can't remember a specific something to attach to, for example, I have to start the whole process over again. It can take me days to answer a simple question like "How did you celebrate New Years' last year?" Needless to say, I usually just choose to not go through that whole process. At all. Instead I have "Now" and "Not now."

Writing this very book you are now holding has been one huge continuous struggle because of the way my brain works. And I am not talking necessarily about the contents of the book. I can always call my parents or talk to Jim if I have a question about a specific anecdote. I am surrounded by reams of paper at any given moment filled with notes of names, places, incidents, time lines, dates, records, and titles. No, the hard part has been deadlines. My editor might say, "Su, I'd like to have Chapter 10 in two weeks, by February twenty-second. Do you think that will be enough time?" I will *always* say, "Yes. Of course!" In reality I have no idea what she is asking and how much time "two weeks" really is. I can look at a physical calendar and count out the days and know that there are exactly fifteen until February 22. But knowing that information, that there are fifteen days until February 22, doesn't mean anything real to me. And then there is another thing to remember on top of that: Chapter 10 is due to my editor in fifteen days on February 22. Now there are two layers of things that I don't understand but that I have to remember and do something about. "Now" and "Not now."

In some ways it's easier for me to deal with these kinds of deficits now that I understand a bit more how the brain works. But the process of becoming aware of how different I am was a very painful one. And the five years from roughly 2003 until 2008 were an eye-opening, heart-wrenching, and overwhelming period of time in my life that leaves me a bit dazed and confused even now.

16

Some Days Are Better Than Others

—U2

For as long as I knew—I always hesitate to say "as long as I could remember"—I kept my truly terrified and genuinely ignorant self concealed, consciously or unconsciously, at least most of the time. But it was an embarrassing and upsetting existence. The ups and downs that I experienced were probably in big part a direct result of the shame and discomfort that I lived with every minute of every day. Just a few years before, I hadn't even been aware of how much I didn't know about the world around me. But at a certain point, I began to realize how clueless I really was. For example, I had trouble remembering my own birthday and how old I was, as well as how old my kids and husband were. I often got lost and was late for classes or appointments, or I forgot about them altogether no matter how many reminders I gave myself or how many calendars I kept. There were days I couldn't tie my own shoes or button buttons. Some days I couldn't read or write. If those happened to be days when I was to volunteer at the school library, read the song list on a spinning CD for a class I was teaching, attend book club or choir, drive to a new pool for a swim or dive meet that required me to read a map and street signs, or even check my kids' homework, then I had to either come up with an excuse why I couldn't, or attempt to fake my way through. This almost always ended badly.

I remember a specific time one summer when I scheduled an annual eye exam for Kassidy on the same day as an afternoon swim meet. Again, understanding the way schedules worked was seldom an area of giftedness for me. Not only were eye appointments with the pediatric ophthalmologist excruciatingly long, they also included eyedrops to dilate the pupils. Sunlight plus dilated pupils equaled eye pain. Swim meets most often occured in the sunlight. Dilated pupils made it extremely difficult, if not impossible, to read (especially maps). That week's particular swim meet was happening at a pool very far away in an area of town unfamiliar to Kassidy and me. I might as well have been in Narnia. There were detailed maps distributed to the kids at practice the day before so that parents and their children could easily find the pool. Parents, that is, who could read maps, and children, that is, without dilated pupils. And Kassidy hated being late for anything. That particular day was a nightmare.

But it was small potatoes compared to the time when I pulled Benjamin out of school during spring of his junior year in 2003.

Though my son was obviously extremely bright, throughout nearly all of his school days he had struggled in the large classes and impersonal environment of public school. And Jim and I had been arguing for what seemed like forever about what to do. Over the years we had looked into the possibility of sending him to one of several small private schools in the area. These schools were highly regarded, as well as hugely successful with kids like Benjamin. Unfortunately, they were also financially way out of reach for us. We lived in an area of the county that had a terrific high school. Thomas S. Wootton High School was regarded as one of the top schools in Montgomery County—for a certain type of student. The type of student that Jim and I both agreed Benjamin was *not.* During Benjamin's 8th grade year—and last year of middle school—I found out about a relatively new public high school in another part of the county that specialized in the arts, both performing and visual. James Hubert Blake High School was one of the three Northeast Consortium high schools in and around Silver Spring, each of which had their own signature programs. They were not a magnet programs per se, so it was initially unclear as to whether or not Benjamin would even be allowed to attend a high school so far out of our cluster. But the bureaucracy that was Montgomery County Public Schools did not deter Jim. He wrote letters to and met with people up as high as the superintendant himself, explaining why Blake High School would be a perfect fit for our son. In the spring before Benjamin's freshman year, we were pleasantly surprised to hear that our request had been granted. Benjamin would be able to attend James Hubert Blake as long as we agreed to transport him the forty-five minutes (one way) to and from school each day. By Benjamins junior year of high school, things were still getting worse academically for him, and Jim and I were really at each other's throat. That is, whenever Jim decided to show up at home. He was still traveling most of the time. And even when he wasn't officially traveling, he worked long hours and most weekends, so that we rarely saw him. Sometimes the only way I knew that he had even been home was by his dirty clothes showing up in the hamper.

I was making Benjamin's bed up with clean sheets on a Friday afternoon early in February 2003 when I discovered a notebook between his mattress and box spring. I pulled it out, opened it, and the writing inside made my heart stop. There were pages and pages of Benjamin's distinctive handwriting: "I hate my fucking life," "I hate going to fucking school with such fucking idiots," "I wish I was dead," "Why does everyone in the world hate me?" "Life Sucks," "Fucking High School sucks," "I want to die!" This kind of stuff, plus lots of other indecipherable scrawls, was written on page after page, over and over again. The entire notebook was filled to near capacity with Benjamin's raw emotion. At that very moment, sitting by myself on his half-made bed totally in shock, I decided that Benjamin was done with the Montgomery County Public School System.

When Benjamin arrived home that afternoon, I told him that I had inadvertently found his notebook, and I held it up. He went immediately into his legendary "Happy Benjamin" patter: oh-Mom-It's-nothing-don't-pay-any-attention-to-that-everything's-fine. I interrupted him and asked him if he would be okay with me making the decision to pull him out of school. He stopped talking and looked at me with such an expression of relief. But not even a minute passed before he looked worried again and asked, "Is Dad okay with this?" Truthfully, I hadn't even thought about whether or not Jim would be okay with it. And frankly, I didn't really care what Jim thought. In my gut, I knew that I had to take my son out of school, or something really bad was going to happen. Like always, I had no plan, but I knew that this was the right thing to do.

The following Monday morning, Benjamin and I marched into the main office of James Hubert Blake High School and asked to speak with Benjamin's administrator. When he eventually appeared, he wished me a good morning and asked how he could help me. I told him that I was there to fill out whatever paperwork was necessary to pull Benjamin out of school. He stared at me with a smile frozen on his face.

I have little recollection of precisely what I said, or what he said, or of what Benjamin may have said, or what exactly happened next. I do recall that at one point the administrator argued that I couldn't pull Benjamin out of school for the simple reason that my son's PSAT scores were among the highest in the school's history. Regardless of that fact, not too long after a fun little powwow in his office, I was filling out paperwork and withdrawing Benjamin from school. Just like that.

Afterward, Benjamin and I went to Checkers and got french fries and milk shakes. When we got home, Benjamin went to bed and slept nearly straight through two full days and nights. On the afternoon of the exact same Monday that I pulled him out of school, he received a letter in the mail informing him that his PSAT test scores had qualified him as a semifinalist for a National Merit Scholarship. When his SAT scores came in the mail later that summer, he learned that he had missed two math questions. Total.

How did I tell Jim about all of this? He remembers a long and intense "dog-walk conversation" one evening. I told him about what I had found (the notebook) and what I intended to do (pull Benjamin out of school). We must have walked those dogs around those soccer fields at least half a dozen times while I talked. Jim also remembers that it hadn't been so much a discussion as my informing him that this was happening. He adds that he hadn't heard that kind of urgency in the tone of my voice, or seen such determination in my demeanor, for a very long time. I'm not entirely sure if he was totally on board with the situation initially, but to his credit, he didn't try to put a stop to it.

Benjamin took his GED exam and (surprise, surprise) got a perfect score. I knew he would have to figure out his next steps at some point. Was he going to get a job? Was he still going to try to get into college? Would he try to pursue acting full-time? I knew he had to figure some of this stuff out, but I also wanted to give him some time to recover. I wasn't sure exactly from what, but I was aware that something was not quite right. We were both traveling through uncharted territory and for several weeks he followed me around like a lost puppy. He occasionally joined my morning classes at the gym, and almost always came with me on the midday dog walk. It was during these long, peaceful walks that he began to open up to me and tell me what school had really been like for him. I was shocked and horrified. Benjamin had been beaten and bullied all through elementary school, middle school, and into high school. He had his PE clothes flushed down the toilet and thrown out of the bus window while in middle school. He always told me he had lost them. He had an English teacher repeatedly "send him to Siberia" when he didn't have his homework. She would have him sit in an unoccupied desk underneath a hanging plant. As he sat there, she would water the plant, and the water would seep through the dirt and stream down onto him. He was often shoved into his locker and pushed off of his seat on the bus. If he was at lunch reading a book, it was often grabbed from him, torn up, and thrown into the trash or a toilet. If it was a library book, or textbook, he told me he had lost it, even when I made him pay for the "lost" books himself. So many dreadful and appalling stories poured out.

I asked repeatedly why he never told me, and he always gave me a similar answer. "Mom, you had enough to worry about." Or, "You wouldn't have been able to do anything anyway." Or, "Mom, you don't understand what it's like at all!" Or, "Telling you would have just made stuff worse." Or, "Mom, what exactly would you have done even if I had told you?" Or, "You don't always do too well in stressful situations." In essence, he was telling me that he had always been more concerned about stressing me out than he had been concerned about his own safety and well-being.

That knowledge was a huge wake-up call for me. The fact was that Benjamin, Patrick, and Kassidy did a better job taking care of themselves, and of me, than I did taking care of them. They regularly took care of me without even thinking about it, doing everything from occasionally tying my shoes and zipping up my coat, to coming to my rescue if I was having trouble with a conversation, to putting up with my "lightning" headaches, my frequent forgetfulness, and my erratic behavior. Yes, I watched and listened to what other parents did and I tried to do a lot of the same "parenting-type" things. I nagged my kids about their homework, I insisted they keep their rooms cleaned up and help out with chores around the house, I bugged them about going to bed "at a decent hour," and I complained when they didn't get up in the morning. If they missed the bus, I drove them to school. If they forgot their lunch, I drove their lunch to school. I did do a million little things for them every day just like every parent does the world over. But the difference was they ended up having to do a lot of stuff for themselves, too, as well as for me. And they probably didn't even think about it. It was just the way it was.

Except it was obvious to me now that Benjamin didn't really think he could count on me, his mother, to be there for him. And he had very good reason to think that. Since he had been a toddler he had somehow understood that he needed to pay attention and look out for me. He was always "a little bit different" in school, in the neighborhood, and to the rest of the family. His grandparents and his aunts and uncles and cousins lovingly razzed him about his excessive talking, his constant questioning, his big confident personality, and the uncontrollable volume of his voice. But in reality it was *me* who was always a little bit different. Benjamin *was* extremely precocious early on. No doubt about that. He tended to push boundaries, he talked (loudly) all the time, he was not afraid to ask questions, as well as declare exactly what was on his mind. *Well, duh!* Of course he did! He had to make sure he knew what was going on all the time! Most of Benjamin's "annoying traits" may have simply been survival skills that had evolved in order to take care of me and, initially, of his younger brother. I am certainly no child psychologist, but it's easy to see how skills like self-confidence, assertiveness, and even his loud, exuberant tone of voice would have had to be developed in order for him to do his job in the family.

Each of my kids, in different ways, formed little parts of their characters and personalities that they could use to effectively look out for me. Patrick is an extremely skillful, patient, and compassionate teacher and coach. The kids he has coached throughout the years, since he was fourteen, in both diving and gymnastics have always adored him and respected him, and their strength and skills have improved under his instruction. I often wonder how many millions of times he had to either tell me or remind me of something or show me how to do something. Patrick is also extremely competitive and can, at times, be fierce, stubborn, and aggressive. I wonder, too, how many millions of times he had to stand up for me even when he was little. And Kassidy. Kassidy can be tough and bossy, but she has always been there, explaining things to me, asking if she could help me with dinner, asking if I wanted to play a game, asking if I wanted to read or watch TV with her, asking if I needed help at the grocery store, and always asking me how my day was. In essence, Kassidy and I really *did* grow up together.

Because Jim was gone most of the time, first the three of us, the boys and I, and then later, after Kassidy was born, the four of us all played together. We read together. We took hikes beyond the backyard, exploring the creek and looking for "quicksand." We sometimes just ate cereal or toast or ice cream for supper. We often laughed together about goofy stuff. There were a million little inside jokes that we shared. We listened to tons of music at the house and when we were in the car going somewhere. We frequently danced around and sang, totally uninhibited. Even Patrick sang along when he was little. As the boys got older, into later middle school and high school, they went off and did their own thing, but they continued to always check in and check up on me. By that time too, Kassidy had stepped in and had started to take over a lot of the responsibility for my welfare. Just as with Benjamin and Patrick, I doubt I knew that she was even doing it, and I doubt she knew she was doing it.

Listening to Benjamin open up and really talk to me on our walks during the spring of 2003 made me realize for the first time how much I depended on him, and in fact on all three of my children. This is the first time that I actively thought about how much *they* did for *me* almost every day. I began to think about how crazy and disorganized and disruptive a mother I really was. Our household rarely had any kind of consistency. As much as I needed and loved daily routine and structure, more often than not I wasn't able to actually bring it off, and chaos often ensued instead. I began to feel absolutely horrible about myself, and the way I had raised my kids. And I began to take Benjamin's battles in school as the thing that proved my point. Maybe not in so many words, but I began to tell myself I had to figure out once and for all how to grow up. Not to *act* like a grown-up, but to *be* a grown-up.

17

Perfect

—Alanis Morissette

As I slowly realized how different I was from other moms, I began to think about and question other aspects of my so-called life. For example, maybe I wasn't really that good of an aerobics or spin instructor. I became obsessed with comments that I heard from members about my classes and compare them with comments I heard about other instructor and their classes. I became overly sensitive to other people's remarks and opinions about the way I taught my classes. I would almost always pay more attention to what one person didn't like about my music, my style, my routine, my shoes, whatever, and less to the twenty or thirty people who loved everything and thanked me for a great class! I started to pay attention to people who left my classes early and to notice when my regulars didn't show up. And I took these things personally. I started cranking out dozens of new spinning CDs, with fresh and often unusual tunes—one-hit wonders from the 1970s and '80s, movie and TV theme songs, music from Broadway musicals, and always an abundance of classic rock! I was constantly trying to be fresh, fun, and original. I started to make my CDs longer, and my classes consequently became longer—and harder. I thought I had to prove myself as the toughest, most demanding, most dedicated, and strongest instructor wherever and whenever I taught. I think I was probably trying to prove how genuine I really was, somehow. Because inside I felt so much like a fraud.

I began to question my marriage. I watched other couples that I knew more closely, and realized that Jim and I were different. Jim was demanding and critical when he was home, and yet he also chose to be away most of the time. I didn't understand how those two qualities could exist at the same time in the family, and in our marriage. How could he want to control everything and yet still want to be gone all the time? Maybe it really wasn't working. Or maybe I wasn't working correctly. Maybe it was me that was the problem.

I also never quite understood why there was never any money. Sure, Montgomery County was an expensive place to live, and I paid to have the kids involved in activities like summer camps, dance classes, gymnastics, swim and dive teams, theater productions, piano and voice lessons. But because I was home, we never had to pay for day care. We didn't take vacations, and rarely ate out. I was careful and watched every dime I spent, cutting out and using coupons for the grocery store, and shopping the sales, the secondhand shops, and clearance racks. Jim had a great job with a six-figure income, complete with corporate credit cards and comprehensive benefits and health care for all of us. I worked only part-time, but pulled in a decent five-figure annual income. Still, when I used my debit card at the checkout of the grocery store, I was often turned away for insufficient funds. Jim would get furious with me if I wrote checks to the school for class pictures, or to the exterminator for our annual termite inspection, without asking his permission. I was often told, "That credit card is dead. Sign this new one and use it instead." There were bounced checks, late fees, and furtive late-night trips to the bank so Jim could "move money around." And then there was the chronic nighttime behavior. Jim was *always* remorseful afterward when I told him about a really bad night in bed. He went to several doctors, tried various medications, and willingly participated in several sleep studies over the years, but he didn't ever get any conclusive answers or reliable treatment.

I talked with my sister Barb with my brother, Mark, and with several of my friends at different times, not about any specifics of Jim's and my situation, but in more of a general way. I was, trying to figure out if what Jim and I had in terms of our marriage was common or normal. I didn't really think so, but a lot of what I thought was often wrong. I was, after all, constantly told how naive, unreliable, and simpleminded I was. I am guessing that my sister, brother, and friends all saw pretty clear answers to my bumbling questions and obvious warning signs in my remarks about marriage and money as I searched for clarification, but nobody ever pushed me to explain further.

About this time, I began to be the Queen of Volunteering everywhere—at church, at the studios and theaters where Benjamin and Kassidy took dance classes and performed in musicals, at the county pool where Patrick dove as part of a national traveling team, at our neighborhood pool where Kassidy swam and dove in the summertime, and at both the high school and the middle school. Many of these volunteer opportunities had an added financial benefit. If I volunteered at the studio, for example, I was offered a significantly reduced tuition for dance classes and performance fees. The ironic thing is, the more I volunteered, the more I worked, the more I tried to be the most perfect wife, financially responsible mother, dedicated parishioner, and best-liked fitness instructor of the entire world, the worse I became at every one of those things.

I had faked my way through my life ever since I had been hit on the head. I acted how I thought I was supposed to act. I did stuff because I saw other people do it. Jim always made his viewpoints very clear to me. I *knew* when I was doing something right or something wrong by the way he treated me and by the way he talked to me. I lived to see his genuine smile and not the scary one. I lived to hear the words "I want to grow old with you" instead "You are always such a stupid frigid bitch!" I desperately wanted Jim's approval, and because of this, when he was home I was nothing but nervous and jumpy, which made things worse, and then he would disappear again on another business trip, or another endless project. So as time wore on I began to take imitation to a whole new insane level. Yet at the same time, I still didn't entirely understand what the rules were for this game of life. The results were predictably disastrous.

18

Hello, Goodbye

—The Beatles

In the fall of 2006, Benjamin was accepted to the American Academy of Dramatic Arts for the January 2007 term. I had never seen him as excited as the day he got his acceptance letter from AADA. Patrick had graduated from high school the previous June, and had accepted a diving scholarship at the University of Maryland in College Park. I questioned Patrick's choice of school, but he was thrilled with his decision and was positively beaming as we moved him into his freshman dorm. Kassidy was a freshman in high school, taking a heavy academic load and continuing to dance every single day.

Jim and I moved Benjamin out to California two days after Christmas 2006. Benjamin had barely been able to contain himself during the weeks and months leading up to this great opportunity, but also didn't bother to start packing anything until Christmas day. My parents came up from Roanoke and stayed at the house with Kassidy, who was not yet driving, and Patrick, who was home, but working and training during most of his winter break.

I had never been to California, and Los Angeles was a bit of a shock. Benjamin's apartment in West Hollywood, which he would be sharing with three other AADA students, was just two short blocks from the campus, as well as an easy walk to Ralphs Grocery store, Target, and a bunch of other shops and restaurants. We shipped his bicycle from Maryland, and he wasn't at all worried about not having a car. "Mom, don't worry! I'll have public transportation around this city figured out in a week!" And damned if he didn't! Jim found an IKEA nearby, and the three of us went shopping and outfitted Benjamin's room with a bed, desk, chair, dresser, file cabinet, and bookcase. To be honest, Jim and Benjamin went shopping. I know I was there with them, but IKEA is one of those warehouse-type stores, like Costco and Sam's, that is so enormous and loud, with so much stuff around as far as the eye can see, and so many people everywhere, that I have trouble filtering; it's all just too much, and I am absolutely lost and frightened. I'm never quite sure if it's a good thing or not, but most of the time I don't remember much about being at places or in situations like this.

The day before Jim and I flew home from California, we went to an official parent orientation and reception at Benjamins school. The president of the school spoke to us, as well as many of the teachers. They told us about the school's history, explained the program, and provided specifics of what was expected of the students, our kids, my Benjamin. It was during that orientation that it really hit me. Hard. I was going to be leaving Benjamin here in Los Angeles, California, more than 2,600 miles away from our home in Maryland. The teachers and administrators didn't know him at all. Nobody at this school had a clue about the way he had always struggled. What if he couldn't keep up with the work? What if he got overwhelmed and depressed and didn't do any work? What if teachers didn't appreciate his incessant talking, and his "expertise" about, well, everything? What if his roommates or the other students didn't get his sense of humor? What if nobody liked him, and he didn't make any friends? What if he was bullied here? I was beside myself with worry. But truthfully, I was really more worried about myself. How was I going to survive without my Benjamin? Sure, I didn't depend on him the same way I used to, to literally help me get through each day without getting too lost. But he had never been so far away. What if I needed him?

~

After getting back from California, I continued to teach aerobics and Spinning classes in the area. I regularly taught ten or twelve classes every week, for the most part at two different Fitness First locations in North Potomac and in Rockville. With the exception of our time in Cairo, I had been teaching at Fitness First Clubs since before Kassidy was born, back when Peter Harvey first started the franchise as Fitness World. I had survived the reigns of numerous aerobics directors and general managers. But as the economy started to slow down in 2006, my job suddenly came under threat. The recession may likely have hit places like health clubs a lot earlier than other areas, and when people tighten their financial belts, it's usually the nonnecessity items that are the first to go. If people have to make a choice between their mortgage and their health club membership, it isn't hard to see why certain decisions get made. I had a huge following of members, who regularly attended my classes, but I was expensive, and I was difficult. I was expensive because I had been working there forever, and those fifty-cent or one dollar raises per class that I earned every year, over fifteen or sixteen years, added up. I was difficult because I was growing up and becoming aware. The aerobics director could easily replace me with an eager, far younger, inexperienced instructor, who would do whatever he or she was told to do, for one-tenth of what she was paying me, and one-tenth of the headaches she spent dealing with me. Game over.

In March (March 8, 2007, to be exact) I was "let go," "taken off the schedule," "fired" (however you choose to look at it) from Fitness First. Before losing this job, I had not realized or actively thought about how much of my *self* was tied up in teaching there. The physical space, the rooms, the equipment, the parking lots, the stereos, the smell, and the Fitness First members were all so familiar to me. I had developed close friendships with many of the people who had taken my classes for years, and I felt suddenly very lost and alone. I became depressed. I had also gotten used to the exercise high, the feel-good endorphins that I'd scored on a daily basis from teaching particularly intense classes day in and day out. It was a huge blow to no longer have that feeling, and I had absolutely no motivation to exercise on my own. I continued to pick up classes at other gyms in the area wherever and whenever I could, but it wasn't the same. My heart wasn't in it, and my confidence was shattered.

There was also something else to think about. And that was

19

Thin Line Between Love and Hate

—Pretenders

I received a phone call from Benjamin just a few weeks after losing my job. His calls always helped lift my spirits, and because he was so talkative, they also helped make my newly endless days go by more quickly. He was always excited about his classes, his friends, his apartment, and his teachers at AADA, and his excitement was contagious. This particular call started out the usual way. I remember talking to him as I walked the dogs. (Those poor dogs! After I lost my job, I walked them *all the time*! I think they both secretly hated me.) Benjamin was going on and on about this, that, and the other thing, and it was a light, comforting kind of chatter. But suddenly, toward the end of the walk as I was nearing our house, his tone changed. "Mom, do you know what myspace is?" Initially, I thought he might be telling a joke: "Do you know what my space is?" It's not always easy to follow Benjamin's train of thought, especially when he is 2,600 miles away. Although I guess I shouldn't really judge. I played along, saying, "No. What?" Then he asked if I was home yet. "Almost, why?" "When you get home go on the computer, and call me right back." Oh, I get it, I thought. Benjamin had recently been finding and sending me funny videos from this new site he had found called YouTube.

When I got home I logged onto the computer, and Benjamin told me exactly what to type and where. I followed his instructions step-by-step, and pretty soon I was staring at something on my screen that was not making any sense to me. There was a site called myspace, and I was reading the words but not comprehending them: "Jim Meck. North Potomac, Maryland. Single. No Children." What was this? I didn't understand. Benjamin awkwardly tried to explain, but nothing he was saying was registering with me. My Jim *was* married. To *me*. And we had three children. This was just some kind of Internet garbage. Right?

I ignored both Jim's myspace page and everything Benjamin told me. He and I didn't talk about it again, and it would be months before I brought it up with Jim.

There was further evidence that my marriage was not exactly on solid ground. Later that spring, I was helping Kassidy look for art supplies for a school project. We kept a lot of extra construction paper, poster board, markers, stickers, and all kinds of additional crafty stuff on shelves in the basement. While searching among the boxes, Kassidy pushed a stack of plastic containers to one side and suddenly an enormous stash of porn magazines and videos tumbled onto the floor. Kassidy and I looked at the floor and then at each other. It was an intensely awkward moment and neither of us knew what to do or say. We both just left the stuff there and went back upstairs. I think I may have found Jim sitting in front of his computer and said something snarky like, "Your fourteen-year-old daughter just discovered your porn supply in the basement." And then I walked away, and I honestly didn't think any more about it. Pornography wasn't something that made any sense to me and it didn't make any sense that it was in our house.

~

My parents came and stayed with us at the end of May. My mom, I think, was worried about me, and even though I was feeling better than I had after losing my job in March, I still felt a little bit adrift. I still had no real plan to speak of. Jim had a business trip out to California that week, and he was planning on extending his stay in order to be with Benjamin on his twenty-first birthday. I was happy to have my parents visiting, and for dinner one night I invited my aunt Sally and Uncle Phil, who lived close by. During dinner, my off-course life came up in the conversation. My uncle Phil said something like, "Why don't you take some classes at Montgomery College?" My aunt Sally immediately agreed. "That's a great idea. Montgomery College has a whole program for people who are going back to school after a long time. You could take a few classes in whatever interested you. No pressure." Uncle Phil taught math and Aunt Sally taught English at the college.

I think I probably laughed at their suggestion, only because I didn't know what else to do. Mom spoke up, and for a moment I thought she was going to save me. Instead she said, "Su doesn't need to go to community college. She went to Ohio Wesleyan and TCU, and probably just needs a few more credits to graduate. But, Su, I think Phil and Sally make a good point. You *should* consider

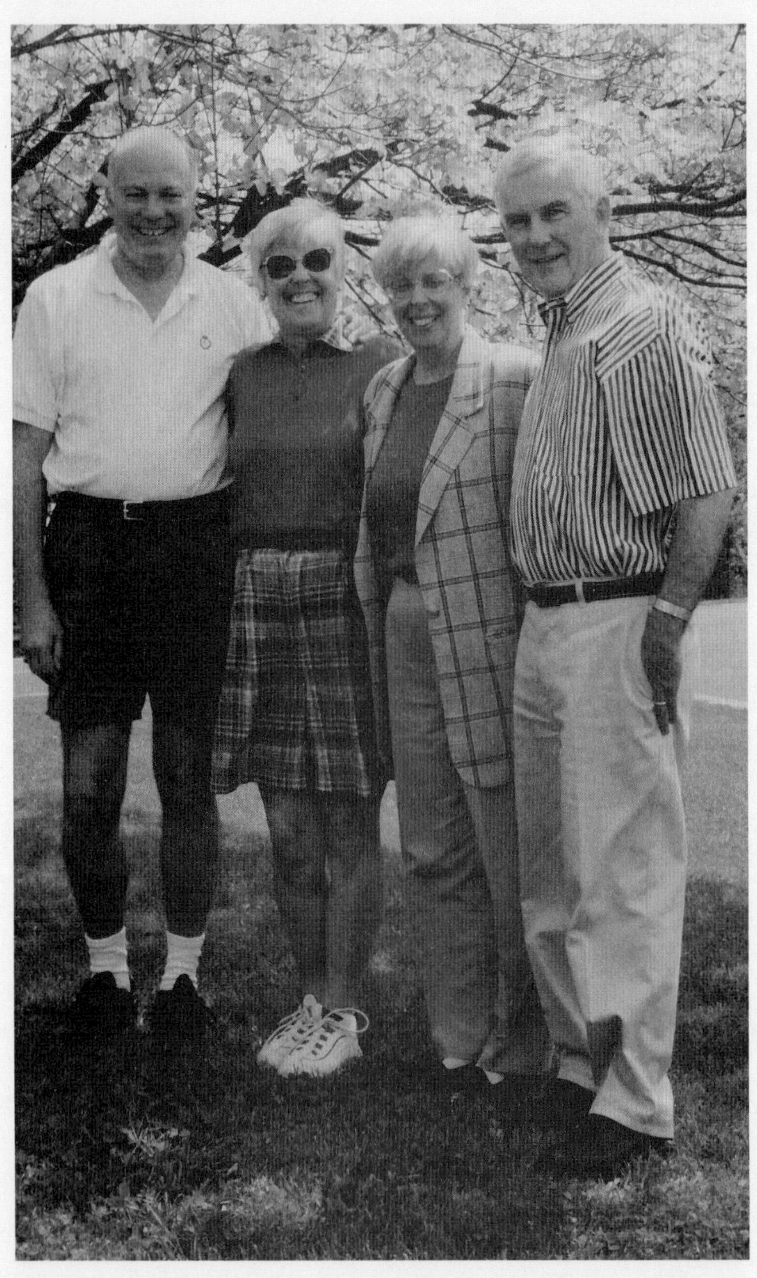

Left to right: Dad, Mom, Aunt Sally (Mom's cousin), and Uncle Phil going back to college and finish up your degree. Now would be the perfect time!" I nervously laughed again, and probably asked if anyone wanted dessert.

The truth was, me going back to college seemed like a totally ridiculous idea. Since my injury, I had never gone to school. I had never sat in a classroom as a student, I'd never written an essay or read a textbook. Going to college, in all likelihood, meant a certain amount of proficiency in math, science, history, English, and who knows what else? I didn't even know all my multiplication tables. It's possible that I had picked up some very basic understanding in a few areas through the years just by listening to the kids talk, and occasionally "helping" them with their homework. But certainly not at any kind of college level! How would I ever explain that to anyone?

Despite all my very real doubts, though, the seed had been planted. When Jim returned from California, I tentatively asked him what he thought about me going to college. Surprisingly, he was all for it, although he agreed with my parents in thinking that Montgomery College would be a waste of time and money. Why didn't I look at American University or Catholic University instead? I went online and looked at requirements for admittance, classes and majors that were offered, and various student activities at both schools. I was immediately overwhelmed, and just as quickly as I had engaged in this little thought process, I dismissed it.

But that's the thing about seeds. If they are planted, they grow. And growing things are often hard to ignore. It wasn't more than a week later that I was logging onto the computer again, but this time I was looking for information about Montgomery College. On an absolute whim, without telling anyone, I drove to the

Rockville campus. I asked directions from at least a dozen people before finding the Student Services Building. I filled out an application, and while standing in line I told myself a million times that I would not be upset if they told me no. When it was my turn, I handed my application to the woman behind the counter. She looked it over, asked to see my driver's license, typed some things into her computer, stamped some other forms and papers, and handed them all to me. I stood there and stared at her. She asked, "Was there something else?"

"Can I go to school here?" I asked. I must have sounded like a total idiot!

"Of course you can, hon. You just need to take that green form and go take a math placement test, and that white form there allows you to take a writing placement test. The pink forms are for you to fill out and send off to get your transcripts from your previous institutions sent here to us."

"And what if I can't do any of the math problems on that test, or I can't pass this writing test?" I held up the green and white papers. I was feeling suddenly very angry. Why were they already giving tests to me before I even went to one class? How stupid is that?

"They're just *placement* tests, hon. You can't *fail* them."

"Oh. Do I do that now?"

"You are certainly welcome to walk over to the Campus Center. The Assessment Center is located on the lower level, and I believe they take walk-ins this time of year."

I knew if I didn't go right away and get this whole testing business over with, I would never return.

I was not at all shocked when nothing on the math test made *any* sense to me whatsoever. What did surprise me was the writing test, or at least the one part that I can remember, where there were series of four maybe five sentences written out. All I had to do was pick the sentence that used the most proper grammar. Since correct grammar is a blood sport in my family, I think I probably did well on that one.

After taking the tests, I was directed to go and talk to Ms. Barbara Gleason, who oversaw the program that caters to the needs of the nontraditional student. Barbara took a look at my math score and suggested a two-week "Fast Track" math program that would be offered later that month. On the evening of June 18, 2007, I entered a classroom for the first time. But even after taking this class every night for two weeks, I wasn't able to catch up and was placed in the most basic uncredited pre-algebra class.

Barbara Gleason helped me pick out two other classes to sign up for in the fall semester, in addition to my math class. She made several suggestions, and I chose a beginning-level sociology class and a health class called Stress Management. I was on my way. And scared to death.

~

But I still had two months left of summer to either prepare for Montgomery College or change my mind. And what a fun summer it was going to be. I wasn't sure what lottery Jim had won, or what bank he had robbed, but he was extremely generous with vacation time and money that summer. Who was I to question that? I thought maybe he was being especially kind to me knowing what a rough couple of months I had had since losing my job. Or maybe he knew how nervous I was about starting school, and he thought I needed a few enjoyable distractions for a few weeks.

In August, Kassidy and I flew out to see Benjamin in California for a week. Jim had seen him in June, but we hadn't seen him since he had left the previous December. Since he started school during the January term, he had classes pretty much all the way through the spring and summer with no long breaks, except for two weeks in August. I couldn't believe he was twenty-one! He looked so great and was incredibly excited to see us! He showed us all over "his town" and gave us a personal tour of his school. We also hiked Runyon Canyon, went horseback riding up by the Hollywood sign, and walked up and down Sunset Boulevard and Santa Monica Boulevard. We all spent a day at a water park as well as a beautiful day at the beach. Kassidy and I both learned a hard lesson about the Southern California sun, which is considerably more intense than in Maryland. We both suffered the worst sunburn of our lives. Which really wasn't the best plan, because immediately upon returning from California, Jim, Kassidy, and I were heading to Ocean City, New Jersey, with my parents for a week at the shore.

While Kassidy and I were away in California, Jim had been tasked with an immediate and crucial proposal order at work that was, unfortunately, about to take over his life for the next three or four weeks. He wasn't going to be able to come with us to Ocean City after all. We were disappointed, but given our sunburn situation, I thought it might just be a blessing in disguise, and I suggested that maybe it was best if none of us went. But Jim said, "Nonsense! My work shouldn't interfere with vacation plans for you and Kassidy. I know how much you guys have been looking forward to relaxing and spending time with your mom and dad. Besides, at this late date, we wouldn't be able to get our deposit back." So it was decided that Kassidy and I would go without Jim. I felt terrible the morning we left. Jim stayed around long enough to help us pack up the car. "My bosses are going to see me and own my ass plenty over the next few weeks," Jim said. "They'll just have to get over me being late this morning. Especially if it means seeing my two best girls off!"

And I was so glad we ended up going. My parents, Kassidy, and I had such a terrific time that week together. We all stayed together at Brown's Nostalgia, a bed and breakfast, just two blocks from the beach. Brown's served delicious four-course breakfasts, and offered homemade cookies every afternoon. There was a huge wraparound porch with rocking chairs to relax on in the evenings. We rented bikes and rode from one end of the boardwalk to the other each morning after breakfast before heading to the beach, where we stayed until late afternoon. We ate out at wonderful restaurants every evening. We people-watched, went to the movies, saw a production of *Seussical* the musical at Ocean City High School, and watched the infamous Twins Contest on the Music Pier. Kassidy and her grandpa rode rides together, and she and I both got our hair wrapped and our ears double-pierced. I talked or texted with Jim every day, and told him how sorry I was that he was stuck at home having to work while Kassidy and I were having such fun. It didn't seem very fair at all.

~

We came back from Ocean City a week before Kassidy was to start her junior year of high school. Jim was in the hospital the entire Labor Day weekend, with inexplicable and excruciating stomach pain and no definitive diagnosis. He was released from the hospital that Tuesday, the day before my classes at Montgomery College were scheduled to start. The night before, I sat on Kassidy's bed and cried. I couldn't do it. What was I thinking? What if I forgot how to read? What was I supposed to do? Despite my Fast Track class during the summer, I was certain that I was doomed to fail as a college student. I found myself asking Kassidy a million questions, like a scared kid.

"What if I don't understand something?"

"Ask your teacher questions."

"What am I supposed to write down? What if I don't know the words and can't spell them?"

"Whatever you think is important write down . . . just sound the words out and write down whatever the teacher writes on the board. If they take the time to write something on the board, write that down in your notebook because it's probably important."

"What if I can't see the board?"

"Sit up front."

"What if I can't find my classrooms?"

"Mom, we just went there this afternoon, and found all your classrooms. We wrote down directions to each class in your new day planner."

"I'm not going. I can't. I just can't."

"Yes, Mom, you can. You're going!"

"What am I supposed to wear?"

"Whatever you want. Be comfortable."

"What if the classroom is too hot or too cold?"

"Take a sweatshirt, and put it on if you're cold."

"Should I wear it, or keep it in my backpack?"

"Why don't you just see how you feel in the morning . . ."

The following morning, I threw up twice before leaving the house. But the important thing was that I did leave the house.

That first semester was incredibly difficult. I had trouble keeping up with all the required reading; I had problems deciphering the notes I took in class. I had questions, but was afraid to speak up in class or talk to the professors during their office hours. I didn't know how to study for tests and quizzes, and I didn't know how to write essays, let alone research papers. I spent hours at home reading assigned chapters over and over again, sometimes the same chapter ten times or more, until I could vaguely understand the ideas and concepts being explained. I battled diligently to work out math problems. Kassidy tried to help me, but part of the problem with math initially was I didn't know my times tables very well, so I spent a lot of time (and paper) adding up numbers instead of multiplying them.

Because I was spending so much time trying to keep up with my schoolwork, a lot of my housework and my usual errands fell by the wayside. The dogs were ignored, and often didn't get walked. Many evenings I didn't cook dinner and Kassidy and Jim ended up having to fend for themselves. I wasn't always able to keep up with the laundry and grocery shopping. Jim was incredibly supportive at first. He called me his "little student," and politely listened to me yammer on and on about my classes and professors. But his supportiveness quickly wore off after a few weeks of soup and grilled cheese sandwiches for dinner. And one night he lost it! "Would it be too much trouble for you to occasionally get off your fat ass and go to the store so we have something to eat in this house? Even if you choose to not eat, I need to." Or words to that effect.

Later that week, I heard him on the phone with a surgeon. He had decided to have a surgical procedure for diverticulitis, a disease of the colon, at the end of October, the same week as my midterms. I called my parents in tears. I couldn't do it. I couldn't go to school *and* take care of Jim and Kassidy. I had only been in school a few weeks and I was utterly defeated. I was tired and worried. I couldn't concentrate, I couldn't sleep, I couldn't eat. I was failing as a mother and as a wife and was failing as a student. Dad and Mom told me to settle down. Of course I couldn't do *everything.* Why was I even trying? They told me my priority should be going to school, and they told me again how proud they were of me for trying. Then they offered to come up during the week of my midterms and help out with me, or with Kassidy, or with Jim, or the dogs.

Knowing my cavalry was coming helped relieve some of my anxiousness for the time being. But I was still nervous whenever Jim was around. I tried my hardest to be done with as much schoolwork as I could by the time he came home in the evenings. I made a point to study for just a couple of hours on the weekends. I skipped a couple days of classes in order to run errands and get the grocery shopping done. But with this new schedule of mine, I was falling further and further behind in my classes, and midterms were looming.

~

On a Saturday morning late in September, everything fell apart for good. I don't remember exactly what the catalyst was, but *kaboom,* I exploded. Jim was sitting on his "big man" chair, Kassidy was sitting on the sofa, and I was pacing back and forth across the family room just ranting and raving about everything that I had kept inside for weeks since starting school. I was trying, if perhaps not very clearly, to explain how hard school was for me, and how unfair it was of Jim to pick the week of my midterms to have elective surgery. Why couldn't he have the operation the following week? Or the following month? I was unhappy that Benjamin was so far away. Why did Jim have to travel so much? Why did he have to work all the time? Everything just poured out randomly. There was no apparent order to my rant, and no real point or purpose. It was just a lot of bottled-up emotion that had to get out.

When I was finished, I stared at Jim. He had been quiet while I had been exploding all over the family room, and now he just said, "If that's really how you feel, I guess we're done." He said it with such a tone of finality. "What? Done?" I was beginning to panic again just that quickly. "Do you mean done with this conversation?" "No, Su. We're *done* done. Finished. I had no idea how unhappy you were with your life with me. I can go and move in with Patrick while we figure this all out." And he walked out of the room. I fell into the elephant chair, exhausted and confused by what had just happened. Kassidy was still sitting on the couch.

"I love you, Mommy."

"I love you too, darlin'."

"Mommy, do you want to watch some *Gilmore Girls*?"

"Sure. That would be great."

The next eighteen hours are a blur. I think there were a lot of phone calls back and forth. Jim called Benjamin and Patrick. Kassidy called Benjamin and Patrick. Benjamin called Kassidy. Benjamin called me. Patrick called Jim. Benjamin, I think, was the one who convinced Jim to settle down and not make any hasty decisions. I think Benjamin also mentioned to Jim that marriage counseling might be an intelligent next step for the two of us to consider.

When Kassidy and I got home from church the next day, Jim called me into the library and said he wanted to show me something he found on the Internet. Instead of going through our health insurance list to find a marriage counselor, he had found a program online. He had been researching it all morning and it looked legit. What did I think? "Sure, why not? How does it work?" Jim pulled up a kind of online questionnaire, and told me that we needed to start with that before we could get any of the other materials. I sat down on a chair next to him in front of his computer. Kassidy was working on her computer just a few feet away.

The questionnaire was set up so we could answer each question independently and then see the other person's answers when we were both done. The questions started out painless enough. What is your partner's favorite color? What is your partner's favorite food? What is your partner's favorite song? Favorite book? Favorite movie? Eventually, they got more personal. How often do you and your partner have sex? How often do you get together with your family? With your in-laws? When was the last time you and your partner went on a date together? Went on a vacation together? Do you and your partner have the same level of education? Do you and your partner both work outside the home? There were about a million questions. The last one was "Have you ever had an affair?" I was happy to be done with my questions, and I was hungry. Jim was done, too, and he asked, "Do you want to do this now?" I looked confused, and he explained that we were supposed to go through each question and talk about them. Jesus Christ! Really? This was going to take forever, and I wasn't sure what could be gained from this exercise. (Silly me!)

We went through the questions one by one. Some we laughed about. (What was the worst present your partner ever bought you? Jim bought me a vacuum cleaner for Christmas one year.) Some we reminisced about. I began to think maybe this was a good idea after all.

When we got to the last question, I showed him my "no." Of course I had never had an affair! Then he showed me his answer, and my world as I knew it ended. He had written "yes." I sat there staring at that word. *Yes.* I was no longer hungry.

20

What If

—Coldplay

On the outside I was calm, cool, and collected. On the inside I was screaming! And I continued to scream for about two or three weeks. I went to class, took notes, asked questions, and screamed on the inside. At home I did laundry, walked the dogs, cooked meals, and screamed on the inside. I attempted to interact with Kassidy the same as always, but I couldn't bring myself to talk to Jim. I avoided even looking at him.

At some point, I called my parents again. I can remember sitting on the bench outside the Theater Building at Montgomery College. I told them what I knew. They told me I could come to Roanoke if I wanted to. Or they could come up to Maryland if I needed them. They said they loved me and that everything would be okay. But how was everything supposed to be okay? How could I get the screaming in my head to stop?

I knew I had to talk to Jim eventually. So I did. One evening I asked simply, "Who was she?"

"Who was who?"

"The woman you had an affair with."

Sigh. "Do you really want to know?"

"Yes."

"I met her online."

So you haven't actually met her? Just online?"

"No. I met up with her when I was on one of my trips to California. She doesn't live too far from Benjamin."

That was how it all started: A simple conversation that proved how stupid, naive, and too damn trusting I had been for so many years. I am staring at the words on the computer screen now. That conversation was just the beginning of what I was to eventually learn about my marriage. Jim ultimately admitted to several affairs that had dated back a decade and a half. And he would tell me more about this affair, which was still going on. And he would tell me the real reason he hadn't gone to Ocean City with Kassidy and me in August: he had flown his lover to D.C. and he had taken her to the ultrafancy Swann House bed-and-breakfast in DuPont Circle. There had been no urgent project that had suddenly come up for Jim at work.

I was to learn where much of our money had really gone for the past fifteen years or so: various strip clubs as far away as Thailand and Canada and as close as Crystal City, Virginia. Strip clubs on Jim's way to visit his family during the holidays. Strip clubs where he went every Thanksgiving when he was in Atlanta. Strip clubs where he offered to take Benjamin and Patrick the one and only time they went with him to Atlanta for Thanksgiving. Strip clubs where he would pay hundreds of dollars for lap dances and group sex in hot tubs. Jim would peruse websites of strip clubs in the various cities he would be traveling to for work, and choose clubs with features, activities, events (and, of course, women) that appealed to him. He would then visit those establishments regularly and pay thousands of dollars to the strippers and dancers that he had handpicked via the Internet. It was so easy! I learned about another woman with whom he had carried on an affair. He paid for vacations, hotels, restaurants, gifts, and plane flights. We were hundreds of thousands of dollars in debt because of years of Jim's "creative playtime." I did not have a dime to show for the years I had worked. He had spent it all, and then some. He had maxed out more than thirty credit cards, some of which had my name, and in turn my credit, linked to them.

Once I became aware of what Jim had been doing all along, I had to know everything. I asked him a considerable number of specific questions about people and places—business trips, money spent, and lies told. And I insisted he answer each and every one. I was beyond angry and beyond hurt, but I still had to know everything. I wanted desperately to understand how and why he had engineered such a double life for himself. I began to refer to every bit of information that he told me as a *shoe* as in "waiting for another shoe to drop." Within just a few weeks, I was waist-deep in *shoes.* After a few months, I was completely immersed. I could no longer breathe because I was buried alive in *shoes.*

Many of the names of people and some of the places sounded familiar to me. Of course they did. These were the people and places of his nighttime rages and abuse. He relived his expensive, degenerate, and brutal, fantasy life with me in our own bed. Lucky me! I had to do something to hurt him. I angrily made a hasty decision and impulsively dug up every single piece of jewelry he had *ever* given to me, including my wedding ring. I found a pawnshop in Gaithersburg, and I made Jim drive me there. I sold *everything* for $350, and told him that I would *never* wear a wedding ring again.

21

Bridge Over Troubled Water

—Simon and Garfunkel

I wanted to hurt Jim like he was hurting me, but I didn't know how. I was feeling a kind of intense pain that was both physical and emotional and it never seemed to let up, even for a minute. I couldn't stop crying. I couldn't eat or sleep. I thought that if only I could get even—if I could somehow manage to cause him similar shame and discomfort—I would feel better. I tried hard to convince myself that I didn't care about anything Jim thought; I didn't want to give a damn about any of his feelings. The notion I had to impulsively sell all my jewelry, for a mere fraction of what it all was worth, in order to upset and outrage Jim, while at the same time helping to make me feel better, turned out to be not such a good plan. And it didn't work anyway. Jim didn't seem the least bit affected by what I'd done and I certainly didn't feel any better. Especially later when it really hit home about how deeply in debt we honestly were. I wished I hadn't been quite so rash.

For years Jim and I had been unknowingly going through cycles. Jim remembers realizing that for most of the time he and I truly existed on "opposite ends of the earth" and he often wondered if he just wanted to be done with me. He talks about how he felt so alone. Jim: "The differences between us had built up so much; created too vast a distance." He would often think about wanting to move out and get his own place. He says now that at any time he could have easily "left me holding the bag" and gone anywhere he wanted. For good. He frequently held that threat over my head. During the lowest points of these cycles, Jim would move his stuff downstairs to the guest bedroom and bathroom, and we would basically try to avoid each other as best as we could.

But this time when he moved downstairs, it was different. I realize now that this was the first time I knew that my marriage to Jim might not be forever. I had always thought that Jim and I were married. Period. And wasn't marriage supposed to be "forever"? But now there was a very real possibility that he could leave me and never look back. I was terrified, angry, and hurt. Plus, having Kassidy around made the hostility we had toward each other all the more awkward.

But Jim says that he eventually thought, "If I was going to try to make it work with *somebody,* why not try—one last time—to see if it would work with you and me?" Eventually, Jim moved his stuff back upstairs. The crisis, as far as Jim was concerned, seemed to be over, or at least manageable.

Because of that, over time there was the slightest feeling of a truce. Several weeks, and then months, passed and eventually Jim and I started talking superficially about household matters: Do you want me to get you anything from the grocery store? Or: If you give me the slip, I'll pick up the dry cleaning on my way in from work. Or: The washing machine is making a funny noise; can you take a look at it? We started walking the dogs together again in the evenings. During those walks Jim would talk to me about people and incidents at work or relay stories he had heard on public radio during his commute. I would tell him about my classes, pass on conversations I may have had with the boys, and tell stories about Kassidy's day. It was an uncomfortable situation, to say the least, but on the other hand, our long shared history couldn't be avoided. Our years of inside jokes, our recognizable quirks and mannerisms, the looks we could give each other sometimes and know exactly what the other person was thinking; all of these things, and more, were impossible to ignore. We started to laugh together again. Although much of what we laughed about was very black humor—inappropriate stuff directly having to do with our current situation. We watched movies in the family room together and afterward we would talk about them. I had never realized before this exactly how many movies dealt with cheating spouses, strip clubs, and lying.

But regardless of how things looked, my rage continued to be right under the surface. I often took out my anger and frustrations on my unsuspecting regulars in my classes at the gym. The littlest things would set me off. If Jim was a half hour late from work, I would think the worst: that he was obviously in bed with someone else. As much as I tried to relax and move forward, I could not. I was constantly grinding my teeth together. I insisted on being on high-alert status all the time in regard to Jim's every word and action. I questioned everything he said or did. I was furious with myself for being so incredibly naive for so many years. For me, forgiveness was not an option and I vowed to myself to never be so trusting ever again. Especially where Jim was concerned.

I can remember a time early the following spring. I was out weeding the beds in front of our house and listening to my iPod. (I *hate* weeding—hate gardening of any kind, really—but this was before I had a really great way to procrastinate and be by myself, i.e., Facebook). My iPod was on shuffle, and songs kept coming up that forced me to think of Jim and me. The good stuff and the bad stuff. I listening closely to the lyrics of songs like Jack Johnson's "Better Together," Postal Service's cover of John Lennon's "Grow Old With Me," Sting's "Perfect Love Gone Wrong," Journey's "Separate Ways," Styx's "The Grand Illusion," 4 Non Blondes' "What's Up," and so many others—one right after the other—for hours as I weeded. I was so angry and confused, but all this music somehow made me feel better. At that moment I just wanted to crawl into a hole with my iPod and do nothing but listen to music for the rest of my life. To hell with anything or anyone else!

I had to talk to someone or I felt like I might burst, so I turned to my family and a few close friends. I had long conversations on the phone with my brother Rob. I told him on more than a few occasions: "Rob, I just want to push Jim down the stairs. . . . I want Jim to be in a horrible car accident. . . . I wish Jim would get bitten by a poisonous snake while he's out mowing the lawn. . . ." Because Rob is super hilarious, he is one of the people in my family that was perfect to talk to when I felt obliged to say such preposterous things. And he understood my rage because he had dealt with troubles in his first marriage. At the same time, Rob is a calm, nonconfrontational kind of person, and although he was always great about listening to my quick-tempered rants, in the end he would usually say something like, "Su, I get it. But you need to take the high road."

For whatever reason, those words stuck with me. I needed to take the high road. I had to be a much better person than Jim would ever have hope of being. I wanted to be able to rise above all of my outrage, hatred, and disgust. But how?

My parents were encouraging me to come and live with them for a time. They told me all about the Horizon Program, a course of study for returning, nontraditional students, at Hollins University, not far from where they live. I drove to Roanoke, and while there, Mom and Dad took me to visit the school. I talked to people at Hollins and had a tour of the beautiful campus. But I didn't get any kind of "wow!" feeling visiting Hollins, and for whatever reason I just couldn't see myself there at all.

My sister Diane also invited me to come and stay with her for a while, which tempted me and would have been tons of fun. When Diane and I get together we are just plain silly, laughing about anything and everything. Diane is also an easygoing, comfortable person to be around as well as being a terrific listener. Our phone calls during this time were epic, and they usually lasted upward of three hours. Living with Diane might very well have lifted me out of my pit of rage and helped me to have a new lease on life.

But I couldn't leave Kassidy during her senior year, and I certainly wasn't about to uproot her! Plus, I was taking classes at Montgomery College and, given our precarious financial situation, I didn't really want to just quit and lose all the money I had paid for not only the classes but also the books and supplies. It's true that I wasn't doing very well in those classes because I was, not surprisingly, pretty unfocused. I struggled more than ever with assigned readings, math homework, and essay writing. But there was a new fierce determination in my spirit that hadn't been there before. I never forgot the extreme anger and contempt that I felt toward Jim. It somehow fueled me to not give up on myself. Ever. Continuing with my path at Montgomery College became my high road.

22

~

Learning to Fly

—Tom Petty

Montgomery College saved my life. That probably sounds superdramatic, but it's the truth. The people at Montgomery College saved me and gave me a life. Yes. That is probably a truer statement. All that, and they taught me how to love learning. And I guess how to learn how to learn—instead of just mimic. When I was learning everything along with my kids as they went through school, I was mostly copying. Copying is not the same as learning. Not that I didn't learn stuff from my kids by copying, but the "reason" piece was missing. The "why am I doing this?" part of learning was missing. At Montgomery College, I wasn't allowed to just copy. I had to show every single step of how I got to the answer of an algebra problem. I had to write an essay explaining why there were advantages in looking at the world through a sociological lens. I had to give an oral presentation about Susan Graham and explain what the mezzo-soprano contributed to the world of opera. I had to think and come up with ideas on my own.

It may sound crazy, but I had never really done that before. Sure, I had made decisions about whether Patrick was sick enough to stay home from school, or what party games we could play at Kassidy's tenth birthday, or whether Benjamin needed new shoes before starting school. I could certainly learn from the decisions I made. For example, Patrick probably should not have gone to school that time he had a temperature of 103 (true story). I learned to take the kids' temperatures and not just see what they looked like before sending them out the door to the bus. And learning from one's mistakes is a good way to learn. Lord knows that I learned most of what I know from first making (occasionally disastrous) mistakes. But making those kinds of decisions and mistakes is not the same thing as *learning* new things.

I learned a lot over the years by simply observing what other people did and what other people said and then doing or saying it myself. But once again, observing somebody doing something or saying something and then doing it or saying it yourself is not exactly the same as learning something. Or at least it shouldn't be. I still didn't understand why I did half the stuff I did. I just knew that it was the right thing to do. I didn't understand why I went to church. But I knew it was the right thing to do in my family. I didn't know why the kids had to do math packets every summer. But I knew that they had them and they had to be completed by the first day of school. I didn't know why I had to make four thousand Christmas cookies every year. But I knew if I didn't my family and the neighbors would ask me why I hadn't made Christmas cookies and I would not have an answer.

But I digress.

The learning I was able to do at Montgomery College had everything to do with me. Not in a gross, selfish way, but in a this-professor-is-here-teaching-his-class-today-and-I-am-a-student-here-to-learn way. And that was new. I was the student who was sitting in that class. I was writing down things in my notebook that I thought were important. Nobody was telling me exactly what to write down. If I wanted something clarified, I had to speak up and ask the professor a question. If I didn't ask, I might never know the answer. I couldn't depend on other people in the class to have the exact same questions I had. This may all sound very trivial and basic, but to me it was *huge!* I was not only learning subject content, whether it be algebra, music history, sociology, or environmental biology, I was also learning to speak up for myself. Nobody was at college with me, talking for me, answering for me, studying for me, writing for me, doing for me. I did stuff by myself. And I learned I was pretty darn good at this learning business. Once I started learning, I just wanted to know more, and more, and more.

But the next fall, Jim said that there was no money for me to continue with school. (Of course there wasn't.) My parents (again) stepped in and agreed to pay for my education, including all my books, until I graduated from Montgomery College. After that, I was even more determined to do well so as not to disappoint my parents. I still wasn't doing it for myself.

Tests made me nervous because I was always worried I wouldn't be able to read or write somehow on the day one was given. Writing papers made me nervous because I had never written them before, and I didn't really know what I was doing. Everyone just assumed that I knew how to research a topic. I didn't. Kassidy held my hand and walked me baby step by baby step through those first few papers. I learned about the Writing, Reading, and Language Center in the basement of the library right before I graduated. Oh, well.

The professors at Montgomery College were there because they loved to teach. Most of my classes there were smallish, no more than twenty or thirty students, and the professors knew the names of their students just a week or two into each semester. The professors were happy to help in whatever way they could. They wanted students to be successful. I don't know why, but I was continually amazed by that fact. Sharon Ward was my environmental biology professor my very last semester before graduating. There was one unit where we had to know how to balance simple equations. I had no idea what that meant or how to do it. Kassidy had enrolled at Barnard College in New York City, so I couldn't ask her for help. I went and talked to Professor Ward and explained that I had never done any of this equation-balancing business before. She sat with me in her office for nearly an hour right then and taught me how to balance equations. Professor Bill Coe was my professor for both pre-algebra and Algebra I. He could probably teach math to a rock, I'm not kidding, and he spent so much extra time with me trying to explain in varied and differing ways how to factor equations. Professor Coe figured out that my basic issue with factoring was that I did not yet know all my multiplication tables. These are just two of the many examples of Montgomery College professors going above and beyond any typical teaching duties, and I will always be eternally grateful for all of the time they gave to me.

But one of the most important things I learned from my professors at Montgomery College was to be honest about who I was and what I had been through. I met Professor Sue Adler at the Awards Assembly for Phi Theta Kappa, the two-year honor society, in the spring of 2008. She mentioned during that assembly that she was the faculty adviser for Phi Theta Kappa, and that students would have the opportunity to interview with her if they were interested in becoming Phi Theta Kappa officers for the 2008–2009 school year. Since I was newly inducted into Phi Theta Kappa, the honor society, I was feeling smart and courageous. I knew those feelings wouldn't last long, so I spoke to Sue during the reception following the assembly, thinking that she would ask me to make an appointment with her. Instead, she said, "Great! Write down your phone number and e-mail for me and I'll contact you as to when our first planning meeting will be during the summer." I guess I was in. That was certainly easy. I loved being part of the Phi Theta Kappa Board, and I grew to love Sue Adler and the other faculty adviser, Brian Baick. Sue is one of those people who only surrounds themselves with other practical and hardworking people. She knows everything about Montgomery College and everyone that has anything to do with the school. She and her husband, Bill, a retired MC professor, are both full of energy and positivity.

It was during my time as an officer for the honor society that I began to open up about the story of my head injury and my journey back to school. Marianne, the group's president that year, wanted all of us to show up at the first planning meeting of second semester with a bag of objects that meant something to us personally, in order to promote a kind of bonding or team spirit among all of us officers. One of the objects in my bag was the Dr. Seuss book *Hop on Pop.* I explained to everyone that the book was the first one I had ever read, and that I was twenty-two years old when I read it. I had never spoken to anyone other than my family and very close friends about any of this, so I have no idea what exactly prompted me to tell these fellow students and advisers the tale. Each person in that room was shocked, and when I finished speaking, everyone just stared at me. I was embarrassed and immediately regretted my decision about saying anything. But I had read their reactions incorrectly. It wasn't "Wow! She's odd." Or, "You poor thing." Or, "Get out of here, you weirdo!" It wasn't any of those things. I don't know what it was exactly, but it wasn't anything critical. And after that, I felt a little less afraid, having gotten it off my chest.

Soon I was telling more and more people my story. After that meeting, Sue talked to Gus Griffin, one of the psychology professors and counselors at MC who specialized in memory. Gus wanted me to come and speak to his class about my injury and my life since. I said yes, simply because I couldn't say no to professors, especially Sue. But I had no idea what I could possibly say to his students. About the same time, Kassidy was enrolled in a first-year seminar class at Barnard all about memory. She told her professor, Alexandra Horowitz, about me, and Dr. Horowitz asked if I would be willing to come to Barnard and speak to that class as well. Again I said yes. Again I hadn't a clue what I would talk about.

I hesitantly approached Jim and told him that I had been asked to speak both at Montgomery College and Barnard about my head injury. I asked if he would be willing to talk to me in greater detail about what happened the day of my accident, my hospital stay, the time when I was first back home—anything, really, that I could possibly turn into some semblance of a speech or presentation. Those first conversations we had were the beginnings of what would become *the* great awareness and appreciation between Jim and me. It became clear at first that Jim didn't have all the facts quite right. For some reason, he thought that my accident happened in the winter of 1988, right after the holidays. And he thought I had been in the hospital for eight weeks instead of just three. But those details were minor compared to everything I did learn from him. And all the things he learned from me too. I ended up speaking to Gus's classes every semester my last two years at Montgomery College. I traveled to Barnard twice to give talks to Dr. Horowitz's first-year seminar. I spoke at my dad's Kiwanis Club in Roanoke, Virginia, and was asked to speak at a meeting of business leaders in Montgomery County.

~

Sue Adler told me about the Paul Peck Humanities Institute scholarship program in the spring of 2010. There were opportunities for students at Montgomery College to intern for a semester at the Smithsonian, the Holocaust Museum, and the Library of Congress. The application process was grueling, but Jim helped me to write out a résumé, and assisted with endless essay revisions. I heard in August that I had been accepted to intern that fall in the music division at the Library of Congress. I could not have been more surprised, excited, and nervous all at the same time.

I started that great adventure right after Labor Day by riding on the MARC train to Union Station in Washington, D.C., and then walking the few blocks to the Library of Congress's Madison Building, which housed the music division. I never got tired of that walk and was always amazed by people who just rushed by the Capitol building, the judicial buildings, and any number of other important government agencies, hunched over their cell phones with their heads down. Uncivil politics aside, Washington, D.C., is an important city, full of significant history. Prominent people have lived and worked there making influential decisions for hundreds of years, and I was awestruck each and every day.

My assignment at the Library of Congress that fall was to help organize and digitally catalog thousands of pieces of Civil War sheet music so they could be seen, accessed, and utilized by anyone in the world. The 150 anniversary of the Civil War was just around the corner and this sheet-music project was to be part of a larger Civil War exhibition. My direct supervisor at the library was Mary Wedgewood. I was a little afraid of her at first because my typing and computer skills were less than adequate for such a task as this. I felt her frustration with me, and that made me nervous. But as time passed I grew to really love and respect her. (And my skills improved a bit too). Mary encouraged me to go to the many varied noontime talks that were offered to library staff, everything from authors, to historians, to scientists, to performing artists, to international celebrities. She invited me to meetings, took me to underground stacks, introduced me to lots of people, and got me involved in the annual Book Festival held on the National Mall. Mary genuinely wanted me to understand that the music division and my single project in that division was just one small part of the history and mission of the library. My experiences that semester were extraordinary.

As graduation from Montgomery Collge approached, I began thinking, What's next? Sue Adler had invited me to roundtable talks with admissions officers from Mount Holyoke College and Smith College. Both schools were small, elite women's colleges in western Massachusetts that had first-rate programs for nontraditional students. Both schools were highly competitive, with rigorous application procedures, but Sue thought I was up to the task. She always had more confidence in me than I ever had in myself. I was accepted to Mount Holyoke College, Smith College, and Columbia University. It was a tremendously difficult decision, but in the end, Smith felt like the right choice.

I received a phone call from Beth Homan, from the Office of Advancement and Community Engagement at Montgomery College a week or so before graduation asking if I would be willing to talk to a reporter from the *Washington Post.* Every year, Montgomery College picked a few human-interest stories to pitch to the news media at graduation time. Daniel De Visé came to our house on a Friday. My parents and all three kids were there for the weekend to help celebrate my upcoming graduation, and thank goodness they were. I don't think I said two words to Dan the whole time he was there because I was so scared about saying something stupid. Jim and Benjamin did most of the talking, filling him in on the injury and my long journey back to school. Matt McClain snapped photos for the forthcoming *Post* article, and let me know that he would meet me the following morning at the college to take more pictures of me on my big day.

Graduation itself was a blur of constant adrenaline. Everything from putting on my cap and gown, to lining up and walking to a huge tent with my fellow graduates, to speeches and receiving my diploma, to pictures, hugs, and congratulations. I can't remember a happier day.

The next day was Sunday, and as I was in the shower getting ready for church, Jim came into the bathroom and said, "You're going to want to take a look at the front page of the *Washington Post* when you finish your shower." My first thought was that the

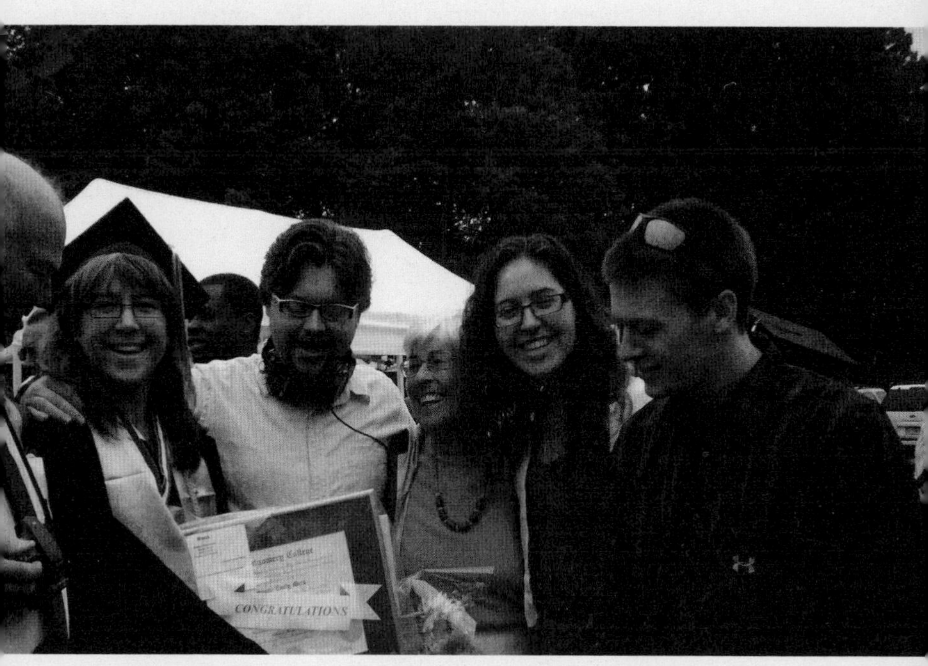

Left to right: Dad, me, Benjamin, Mom, Kassidy, and Patrick at my graduation from Montgomery College, May 2011

United States had endured another terrorist attack. Imagine my surprise when I squinted to read the headlines. I grabbed my glasses and looked again. There I was on the front page of the *Washington Post*! Holy shit! Dan had written the most amazing, heartfelt piece, and I was instantly in love with the man and his ability to make words sound so perfectly put together.

Dan's *Washington Post* article led to a BBC interview, a radio interview with *Elliot in the Morning* on DC101, and a spot on the *Today* show. All of that led me to Peter Steinberg, a literary agent in NYC, who helped Dan and me write up a proposal for this very book. Peter then helped me through what seemed like a million meetings with different publishing houses in New York to see what kind of interest there might be about a story such as mine. From Dan's article to the signing with Peter and everything in between—it all happened in a matter of a few weeks.

It was a whirlwind of feverish activity, compounded by the fact that our house was on the market and we would be moving to Northampton, Massachusetts, that summer in order for me to start at Smith College in September. Life is never dull!

23

Wish You Were Here

—Pink Floyd

Monday, June 20, was just another hot and humid day in a long string of hot and humid days in Gaithersburg, Maryland, during the summer of 2011. I slept in a bit that morning, and by the time I finally walked Lucy and Linus, the summer swelter had surged past ninety degrees. After just half an hour, and only half of our regular walk, the dogs and I had definitely had enough, so we turned around and trudged home. While Linus chomped away on "ice treats" on the cool floor, I got myself a huge tumbler of ice water and sat down at our kitchen table to check my e-mail on our Mac laptop. Jim was working out of the house by this time, preparing for our move to Massachusetts later in the summer, and had come up from his basement office to grab an early lunch.

As a result of all the media attention my story had gotten, I had been flooded with e-mails and Facebook friend requests from far and wide. There were a few weirdos, but for the most part people simply wanted to offer their support and share with me their own stories of personal struggles. I often felt humbled as I read what people sent, and I tried my best to respond to everything that came to me. On this particular morning, as I scanned a dozen or so new friend requests, one in particular caught my eye. It came from a "Neal Moore." The name sounded vaguely familiar, so I clicked on it, but there was no picture and not much information on his rather anonymous Facebook page. I immediately thought weirdo, but at the same time I was certain I had heard the name before. So I asked Jim if the name "Neal Moore" meant anything to him.

"Sure," Jim said. "He was your high school boyfriend, the guy you were seriously dating when I met you." At Jim's words, I suddenly recalled Neal's name occasionally coming up when Jim tried to tell me about my life—our lives, really—before he and I had met. I also vaguely remembered my parents talking about a Neal in some remote conversations. And then yes, I was sure I had heard some mention of a former serious boyfriend by the few high school and college friends with whom I had reconnected over the years. I told Jim that Neal had contacted me on Facebook, and I asked if he would have a problem with my accepting his friend request. Jim just laughed and said, "No . . . Why would I?"

What happens when most other people get Facebook messages from long-lost boyfriends or girlfriends? Maybe there is a sudden flood of various emotions? A rush of warm, sweet, familiar pain in the chest? Possibly a surge of significant memories—vivid images of long, sweet kisses in doorways, of hushed late-night conversations on the telephone, of bodies coming together lovingly under crisp sheets? Or maybe instead there are overwhelmingly less favorable emotions: jealousy, resentment, anxiety, or insecurity.

I, of course, didn't get any of those feelings, sensations, or emotions, good or bad. Neal wasn't an actual, flesh-and-blood memory to me. He was simply another character in another set of stories I had been told about. I had absolutely no real recollections of Neal, no emotional investment in our earlier relationship whatsoever. Was this "Neal Moore" my first real love? Friends and family assured me that he was, but what did that matter, if all trace of that love had been wiped from my memory? But then I began to wonder. There had been a point when I hadn't remembered my parents or my brothers and sisters. There had been a point when I had not had any vivid images of my kids. There had been a time when I had no real feelings for my husband. And yet the expectation, and eventually the reality, was that I loved all of these people. Was this really any different? Neal and I had loved each other passionately in some kind of previous life. That was a fact. And the facts kept coming.

Already, fate had delivered me two previous chances to reunite with Neal, and I had failed to follow through either time. The first chance was a decade ago, when I was visiting my old friend Kathy in Pennsylvania, near where my family once lived. "We got in the car and went for a ride," Kathy recalls. "You wanted to see the house you grew up in, in Chesterbrook. We went and looked at your house, but you had no recollection of it. Over the course of our conversations about the good ol' days, I said, 'You know, maybe Neal is in the phone book.' " I had no particular reaction to that thought. Entirely on her own initiative, Kathy dug out a phone book, pawed through it, and found a listing for Neal's family in Phoenixville, the suburb where Kathy, not I, remembered his family had lived. She wrote down the number on a sheet of paper and handed it to me; she seemed excited at the prospect that I might call him. I didn't. I don't know why. Maybe I wasn't ready yet. I kept that piece of paper with his family's phone number on it stashed at the bottom of my underwear drawer.

The second chance came years later, when I was in Pennsylvania again, this time on a college-looking trip with Kassidy. On this trip, I met up with an old friend from my high school marching band drum line, a man named Lenny Brown. Lenny had friended me on Facebook months before, and I messaged him that I was going to be in Wayne for a day or two with my daughter, and did he and his wife want to meet to catch up? Lenny and Mary met us at a restaurant in King of Prussia. We talked, and Neal's name came up again. When I returned home, I mentioned Neal to Jim. Jim remembers saying, "Well, Su, we can probably find him if you want. And we got so far as a phone number and e-mail address. And I thought you had initiated it then." I hadn't. I don't know why. I guess I still wasn't ready. But I printed the records from the computer and kept that information in the same drawer.

But this situation was different: This time, Neal had contacted me.

~

I really had no idea what I was starting when I wrote my first message to Neal. Hell, I didn't even know for sure if this was the same Neal Moore I had dated almost thirty years earlier. Neal Moore. It's not such an unusual name; and of course I kept thinking the author of this friend request, with his anonymous Facebook page, might be nothing but another weirdo.

Late in the morning of June 20, I wrote: "Are you the Neal Moore that I have heard about for so many years? If so, I would love to talk to you at some point and have you fill in some gaps." That was a generic enough reply, I thought. There was a lot I didn't know about my time in high school. The tales I always heard about my school years before going to college at Ohio Wesleyan were full of wild pranks, drunken incidents, long stretches of dark emotional moods, and constant battles with my parents. Certainly nothing very positive was ever related to me. Would Neal, if he was the Neal of my youth, just have more of the same?

I held my breath.

A reply came two days later: "I don't know what you've been told or not told about me, but to answer your question in a word, yes. I can't believe it's really you!" I was about to learn a lot more about Neal, and a lot more about myself. Remember, at the moment I made contact with Neal, the sum of my knowledge of my three-year relationship with this man would have fit into this one single paragraph.

A week earlier, Jim and I and my amnesia had all been guests on NBC's *Today* show. An old friend of Neal's watched the show, heard my story, and noted the odd spelling of my name. Neal recalls: "She e-mailed me and said, 'Did you watch the *Today* show this morning?' And I said, 'I never watch the *Today* show.' And she said, 'Well, you might be interested in this, because I think I saw Su as a guest.' And I said, 'It can't be, because Su died in a car accident twenty years ago.' "

~

Neal and I had dated for three years. Then the relationship had mysteriously evaporated. Then I had died—or so Neal thought. Losing me had pushed Neal into a sort of hibernation. For the next few years, he threw himself into work and study, moving out of his parents' home and living in solitude, avoiding old friends and new girlfriends. His parents feared for his health. It was the first time since the start of high school that Neal wasn't attached.

From Neal's perspective, our relationship had lacked a proper ending. When I left for college, we were all but engaged. We had a wedding date, if only in our own minds. And then Neal had visited me at college and found me distant and kind of standoffish with him. When I returned home after just one trimester for winter break, I was in an unwavering, unreadable sulk.

"Christmas break we were together," Neal recalls. "It was initially tearful. You were upset. I was upset." It was on that visit, apparently, that I told Neal about Jim. "You just put it out there as somebody you met at school, and you were dating him there, but when you were with me, you wanted to be with me." After the break, I went back to school and Neal recalls, "We continued on like nothing had happened. During the following summer when you were back home and working at Picket Post Swim and Tennis Club, I thought everything was back to normal with us. Because it was. And then your letters stopped coming abruptly during the end of your second year at school."

The following year, 1985, Neal ran into one of my friends. She told him a wrenching story: "You were on a highway near Delaware, Ohio. You were coming home from a weekend, or something like that. You were passing a tractor trailer, and you came out around it, and it was a head-on collision. I remember sitting on the edge of my parents' bed in their bedroom and telling them." My parents had moved away by the time Neal heard about this, so he had no real way to check the story out. In those pre-Internet eighties, he could find no obituary, no record of my passing. And of course by then I was no longer Su Miller. I married Jim in May of 1985, and was now Su Meck.

Back in the present, Neal's friend persisted: "The name is Su Meck, but it's *S-U,* like Su used to spell it, and this woman looks just like Su, only older." Neal sat in his office at work that morning and searched online for the *Today* show video. He found it and clicked on the link.

Neal recalls: "A woman I work with came into my office and said, 'What's the matter? You're white.' And she sat and watched it with me, and she said, 'Is that the girl you talked about?' Anybody who knows me knows about Su. And she said, 'Well, she doesn't look dead.' And pretty soon all the women in my office were watching this recording with me. And they were all like, 'Contact her, contact her!' And I didn't know how to contact you."

Neal found me on Google first. Then he opened a Facebook account and dispatched his first friend request on June 20, 2011.

After getting past the initial surprise that I was indeed the long-lost, ex-dead girlfriend, Neal and I fell into a comfortable Facebook relationship, swapping stories about our current family situations, kids, spouses, careers, music, and hobbies in an effort to become reacquainted. Neal told me he was married with two children. He and his family were living near his childhood home outside Philadelphia, and he was working as CFO at a company that provides video on demand for hotels and resorts. I told him I was married with three grown children. The domestic revelations cleared the air of any potential romantic tension.

~

Reconnecting with anyone who knew me before my injury has always been especially tricky for me. My behavior typically follows a predictable pattern: I remain cheerful but noncommittal as I unconsciously work constantly to figure out what the expectations in this relationship are. Then, also unintentionally, I labor to mold myself into whatever person I can be to fulfill those expectations and make the other person "happy." This is never entirely fair to me or to the person I am meeting. I know that. But I still do it, and I don't even realize what it is I'm doing until I stop and think about it much, much later.

With Neal, I made an effort almost immediately to direct our conversations into the past. I wanted to hear how we first met, if we had known each other before dating, if he had graduated from Conestoga High School, how long we dated, what kind of stuff we did together. I had nothing but questions for this poor man. In my first messages to him, I downplayed the shock of rediscovering such a major character from my long-lost past. But inside I was jumping for joy! Here was a person who just might be able to fill in countless gaps from that time and answer innumerable questions. Neal had absolutely no reason to lie and no motive to try to protect me. I got the feeling almost instantly from him that if I asked him a question, he would be most liable to answer me straight, without any spin. Neal Moore could conceivably be a terrific source of valuable information.

Neal told me about my car accident. I replied with a smiley face, "I was not killed in a car crash . . . just hit with a ceiling fan." Incidentally, I found out when writing this book that Jim and I were in fact in a car accident on our way to Cuyahoga Falls for a weekend family gathering late in the fall of my sophomore year. Jim had invited me just to get off campus for the weekend. During that accident, my head had hit the windshield of Jim's Malibu, and I had been taken to the emergency room. Jim's car was smunched, and I had a fairly serious concussion, but I certainly hadn't died.

Then Neal began to fill in the many details and exact particulars of our long ago romance. He was a projectionist at the cinema and a teller at a bank; I was a lifeguard at the swim and tennis club in my family's neighborhood of Chesterbrook. He was older and had graduated from Phoenixville High School but he had agreed to take me to my Conestoga homecoming dances and proms. We spent summer days, when we weren't working, at his family's pool. I would write him little notes and decorate them with hearts, stars, and doodles. I told Neal that sounded so "girlie." No, he said, I was more the "romantic tomboy." He said he had a box filled with graduation pictures, prom pictures, and letters I'd written him, but all of it had been destroyed four months earlier in a basement flood. Very bad timing.

We traded our first messages on the morning of June 22. By that same afternoon, we were already joking around and feeling remarkably comfortable with each other. Neal declared, "I'm always here for you!" I wrote, "I don't know if it would ever happen, but it would be nice to meet you someday :)" Neal replied, "You already have met me, but perhaps a reunion one day would be nice."

That night, I asked my parents about Neal. My mother said, "Oh, that Neal Moore! He really straightened you out!" She recalled that I was "so much better behaved" after we started dating, and that I would often listen to Neal when I wouldn't listen to them or to anyone else, even if he and my parents were telling me the same thing. Mom then recounted a story from the end of my senior year as an example. Apparently, I didn't want to go to the Conestoga High School baccalaureate service, undoubtedly because I thought I was way too cool for something as stupid as that. My parents were insisting that I go, but I kept refusing. (Most likely I was refusing simply because they were insisting.) According to Mom, Neal came in and announced that if I didn't go to baccalaureate, he wouldn't take me to the senior prom. He told me I would regret it later if I didn't participate in all of the senior events with the rest of my graduating class. He even offered to go to the service with my parents and me. (For some reason my mom asked me if Neal still had his Jeep. Really, Mom? I doubt he had the same Jeep after thirty years.)

Dad mentioned that he thought he could dig up some slides of the two of us, if I was interested. I was very interested, particularly since Neal had lost all of his pictures, as well as all the letters and all the other paraphernalia from the "Su and Neal" years. The only items he still had were a pencil portrait that he had drawn of me in his sketchbook—from my senior portrait, because I would never sit still long enough to be sketched; an Ohio Wesleyan sweatshirt; the Cabbage Patch Kid I had presented him at Christmas one year, which we had playfully named Arthur Miller-Moore, and a few mix tapes hand-lettered by the teenage me.

For me, our reunion meant the recovery of another lost chapter from a forgotten life. For Neal, my very existence set off a sort of existential time bomb. "I didn't know how to feel," he recalls. "I had put it in my mind that you'd been gone all these years, and all of a sudden you're here again. It tore me apart, to be honest."

Neal's years with me had been "one of the happiest times in my life," he recalls. "We saw each other or at least talked to each other on the phone every day of our lives from the day we met. I

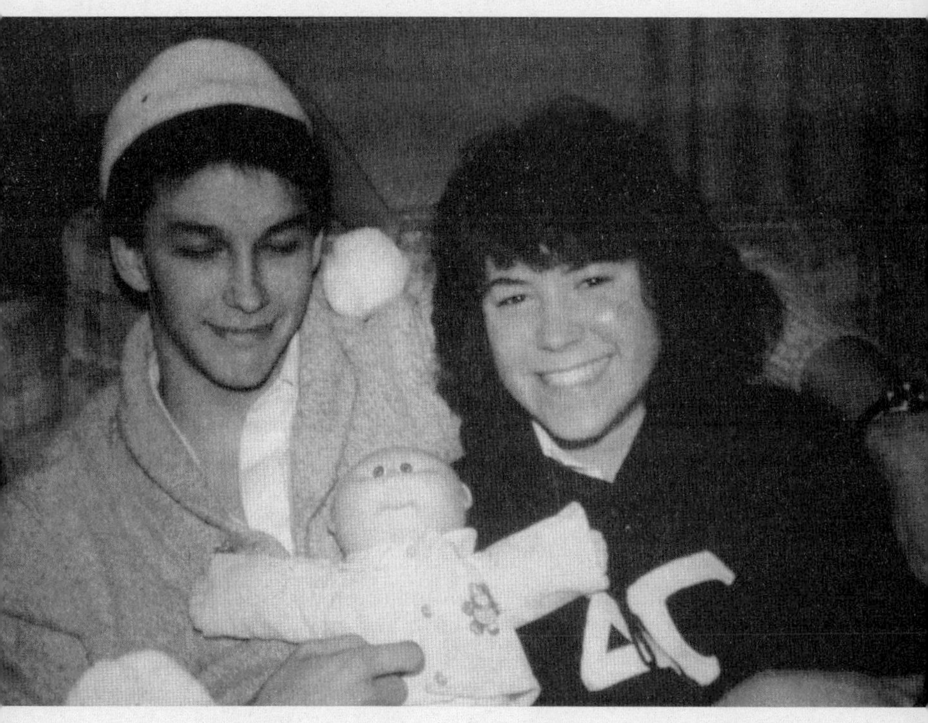

Me and Neal Moore together at Christmas after my first semester at Ohio Wesleyan. For Christmas I gave Neal a Cabbage Patch Kids doll that we named Arthur Miller-Moore because we had seen the movie *Arthur* on our first date.

had had many girlfriends in high school, but what you and I had didn't even compare to that."

I was needy, I was directionless, and Neal was my compass. He remembers me as the Jan Brady of the Miller household: "You were one of the ones in the middle. I won't say that you were put aside or neglected—your parents would never have done that—but you felt that way. And I gave you the attention you craved. You could have had any guy in school. You had a lot of male friends. But you never attached to anybody. You were one of the guys. You were a tomboy. That's what attracted me to you, because you weren't the same kind or type of person I was used to dating, girlie girls who were boring. We used to go out to Valley Forge Park and get dirty and sweaty while hiking." Our favorite bands were the Who, Pink Floyd, and Queen. Our favorite Who song, Neal remembers, was "Bargain," from their 1971 album *Who's Next.* With Queen it was "You're My Best Friend" and "Fat Bottomed Girls." And with Pink Floyd, probably the title track from *Wish You Were Here.* Neal told me I wrote *Pink Floyd* and *Neal Moore* all over my sneakers when I was in school. Later on, he would tell me how I lost my virginity with him at Valley Forge Park. "I didn't push it," he recalls. "One day after we had been dating for nine months or so, you just came to me and said, 'Let's go have a picnic.' We went out for a walk and a little picnic, and you just turned to me, and one thing led to another. There were no words."

Every year for the past twenty-eight years, Neal has driven to Valley Forge on September 17 to mark our "first date" anniversary. He walks along old hiking trails that he and I had hiked together, and remembers what was. It is a sweet and yet heart-wrenching tradition. I try to grasp what Neal tells me, and understand that tradition, but I never will completely appreciate his September 17 ritual simply because Valley Forge Park is just a tourist destination to me.

~

In a Facebook exchange on June 24, 2011, two days into our new relationship, I told Neal how nervous I had been during the *Today* show interview. I wrote, "I hate when people ask, 'What is your first memory?' I just want to ask them what *their* first memory is!" Neal replied, "OMG! This is the first time since we reconnected that you really sound like the girl I used to know! I love it!"

It was the first time anyone from my old life had ever told me I sounded like the old me. Was Neal saying it merely because he wanted me to be the same girl? Was he living a fantasy, imagining me as a perpetual eighteen-year-old? Or did he really think that I was the same person now as then? I have to wonder what he would have thought if we had reconnected ten years earlier. Back then, I had very little sense of humor, and I mostly just parroted things other people said. I didn't think for myself then. I do now. Or at least more than I used to.

We began sharing more details of nearly three lost decades, and Neal ticked off an ever more impressive list of accomplishments. "We have lived in Edinburgh, London, Paris, Amsterdam, Prague, Sydney, and Honolulu," he wrote, but "Monte Carlo is my favorite place in the world." On his fortieth birthday, Neal and a friend went heli-skiing in New Zealand. Neal has climbed Mount Kilimanjaro. He knows enough of seven languages to get around. He was once head chef at a three-star restaurant.

Though he probably didn't mean it, Neal and his stories were starting to make me jealous. He was so successful, so well traveled, such a great father, husband, and chef, while my life has felt like one battle after another, and my kids subsisted mostly on mac and cheese. The more I heard about Neal, the more I wanted to know him, and to see him. Was he leading me on? Was this old boyfriend too good to be true? Can a person really be that sweet, successful, and smart?

If Neal wanted a reaction, he got one. On June 25, three days after our first message, I had lunch with an old friend from high school. I told her about Neal. At the mention of his name, my friend turned white, looked surprised, and just stared at me for a moment. Then she caught herself and tried to recover as she told me that, yes, she had some vague memories of him. I threw the bullshit flag, sensing there was something she wasn't telling me. She sighed and began to confess. She proceeded to tell me a story that would change my life. Again.

~

In fall of 1983, I left for college very much in love with Neal Moore, much to the chagrin of my girlfriends, some of whom were still in high school at Conestoga. They didn't like Neal, because I wasn't nearly as "fun" or "crazy" since I had started dating him. It seemed they thought I would be missing some kind of "Total College Experience" by keeping a serious boyfriend, especially someone like Neal, back home. They took it upon themselves, if not to break us up completely, at least to drive a wedge into our relationship. One of these girls wrote to me at college and told me that Neal had been seen with an extremely attractive young woman at the King of Prussia Mall. When approached, Neal had supposedly blown her off and told her that if Su had gone all the way to Ohio, he could do whatever he damn well pleased back in Pennsylvania. Upon hearing this story, I got really fired up, distraught, angry, hurt. I was totally pissed off. Seizing on my agitated state, one of my friends—my lunch date, in fact—had dared me to sleep with someone at college, anyone really, just to get back at Neal. That guy turned out to be Jim Meck.

Listening to this story and letting it sink in, I was, on the one hand, sort of amused, thinking back to how young and juvenile we all were. I really was quite the gullible innocent. On the other hand, the more I thought about it, the more I began to get angry. A week earlier, this new narrative wouldn't have mattered, because I had no stake in my old relationship with Neal. But in my new reality, the tale took on tragic proportions. Over the course of a few days, I had learned, first, that Neal just might have been the love of my life, and, second, that our love had been stolen from us by jealous teenage girls. My so-called friends changed the course of my life with one silly, adolescent prank. That sounds overly dramatic, I know. Who really knows if Neal and I would have survived four years of a long-distance relationship in the eighties, before e-mail, cell phones, texting, Facebook, and Skype? But I guess I would prefer to know for sure, and now there is no way to know.

That evening, I wrote to Neal. "I just learned today about some very interesting facts about what REALLY happened in 1983–1984 and I am REALLY pissed off!!! It amazes me how people (my so-called best friends at the time) can lie and alter the course of someone's life . . . and get away with it for twenty-five-plus years!!!" The explosion of capital letters and exclamation points caught Neal off guard. "Calm down," he wrote. "Let's talk." Then he vanished from cyberspace for a full twenty-four hours; maybe I had scared him off, or maybe he just needed time to think. When he resurfaced, he seemed to share my sense of loss.

"I'm feeling a lot of emotion as things are starting to sink in," he wrote. "And, like you, I'm pissed off because it doesn't seem like we even had a chance . . . And there never was anyone else but you. Ask my mother, who kept telling me to let you go and move on." As Neal processed the new information, the end of our relationship began to make more sense. "There were sooo many questions left unanswered that have plagued me over the years," he wrote. "Honestly, there hasn't been a week that has gone by that I haven't thought about you. You really set the bar for all of my relationships since . . . You weren't just a girlfriend/lover, but my best friend, and I kept kicking myself as to what went so wrong that we were torn apart so abruptly. We were, at one time, inseparable."

In some ways, I don't know what happened to Neal and me, either. I wasn't dating Jim then. I had just slept with him once to get back at Neal. Why did I not say any of that to Neal at the time? Why didn't we talk until we got to the bottom of the situation then? Did I just feel too overwhelmingly guilty? Was I just too afraid of losing Neal altogether?

~

I have trouble with virtual reality in the sense that if I haven't actually previously met somebody who happens to be on the other end of a phone, or e-mail, or text message, that person isn't "real" to me. It's hard to explain, but since I had never met Neal in person, he is no more real to me than Santa Claus, Jesus Christ, or the tooth fairy. He sent me a few recent pictures, but unfortunately I still haven't been able to wrap my head around Neal as an actual person. Instead he has, in my mind, been a sort of pen pal, an unknown entity "out there" that cares for me somehow. We talk and text, telling each other stories and helping each other through crazy things that happen in our lives.

"I'm sorry for saying what I am going to say next," I wrote Neal on June 27. "I REALLY want to meet you!!! It doesn't make ANY sense . . . but there it is!!!" For weeks after that I sent messages, pushing to meet him before we moved to Northampton in August. Neal resisted. "I have three fears in eventually meeting," he replied. "They are, in no particular order, (1) disappointment that I look older, (2) all your memories come back and you are more angry as to what happened, and (3) no memories are triggered."

I have never fully understood Neal's reluctance to meet. Those fears seem so ridiculous to me. How could he possibly look "older" to me? And as far as memories coming back or not, I have kind of given up on that whole scenario. I have had my hopes raised and then dashed too many times. But I have fears of my own: Maybe Neal has a picture in his mind of Su the eighteen- or nineteen-year-old, and, let's face it, I am now 48, and really quite a different woman from the one he remembers. Maybe he's secretly worried he would be disappointed with how I look now, or how I act, and he wants to preserve me in his mind as a youthful fresh-faced teenager.

Neal sent me a picture of himself as he looks today. I messaged him as I opened it: "I am staring at your face, trying so hard to remember . . . but there's nothing. I hate this SO MUCH!" Neal seemed to think that seeing his face would trigger a cascade of old memories. I knew better. I told Neal he had a kind face. He shot back, "Santa has a kind face." I found that funny, because in my mind he was as unreal as Santa. But I didn't tell him that.

For various reasons—time, distance, our separate families, and busy lives—Neal and I have still never met. But we text often and have spoken on the phone maybe a dozen times. It was awkward at first; I have trust issues, particularly after learning all of Jim's transgressions. I wanted to know if Neal was for real. "You didn't trust me," Neal recalls. "You said, 'How do I know it's you?' And I said, 'You have this scar.' " And he described the scar on my abdomen that I have from a stupid adolescent incident in Ocean City. I was beyond shocked. How could this man I'd never met have such knowledge of my body? I demanded, "How do you know that?" Neal said, "I know every inch of your body."

Our first conversation was weird and wonderful for both of us. Strange for him because he said I sounded the same as I did when I was eighteen, just as he remembered, and strange for me for the opposite reason; because I didn't remember him at all. During this phone call, he told me about our first date. It is a story I never tire of hearing.

≈

It was September 17, 1981, and a friend of mine who was dating one of Neal's coworkers at a local movie theater set me up with Neal on a blind date. It was the beginning of my junior year in high school, and I was sixteen. I should interject here that I had never really dated in high school. I had a big group of friends with whom I hung out and partied, and because I was a drummer in the band as well as a bit of a jock and a tomboy, I had lots of close guy friends. But not boyfriends, specifically. It brings to mind my mother's words: "You had only two serious boyfriends in your life . . . Neal and then Jim."

On that September evening, Neal arrived at our door, and, in his recollection, "your parents hated me right away." He was three years older than me; he had just turned nineteen, and he had flamed out of Penn State the previous year. He was living with his parents, but working as a teller in a bank in Philadelphia, and also working at the movie theater so that he could pay for night classes at West Chester State. I seriously doubt my parents hated him—but that's how he tells it.

We met my girlfriend and her boyfriend outside the theater. We all went in, purchased huge buckets of popcorn, and proceeded to find seats in the auditorium where we sat and watched the movie *Arthur.* Who knows why, but we became a bit rambunctious during the movie and began throwing popcorn at each other. Neal says there was popcorn everywhere—in our hair, down his shirt, all over the seats, and on the floor. He told me that, to this day, he still cannot eat popcorn without thinking of that night. He also recalls thinking during the date that I was "way out of his league," whatever that means, and he thought this would be our one and only date. We exchanged phone numbers, but he never expected to hear from me again. He did not kiss me good night.

The next day was a Sunday, and I had gone to the library to do some homework. As I opened my purse to get a pen, popcorn came tumbling out onto the table where I was working. I laughed out loud. When I got home, I called Neal and asked if he wanted to go for a walk in Valley Forge Park. After he got past the astonishment that I was really calling him, he agreed to a walk, and he drove down to pick me up. We headed to Valley Forge, parked the Jeep, and began walking on the path that winds for miles through the park. Neal recalled that we were "just talking together about everything." At some point, I turned to him and asked him straight out, "Why didn't you kiss me good night last night?" He said that's what he eventually grew to love about me, my straightforwardness. He said he always knew where I stood; I didn't play games, although I did enjoy pushing limits. Apparently, I didn't even wait for him to respond, I just planted a kiss squarely on his lips. He remembers initially being taken aback, but there were quite a few more kisses on that Sunday afternoon.

It sounds like we spent quite the enjoyable first weekend together. And though I love my family more than anything, part of me will always wish I had been there.

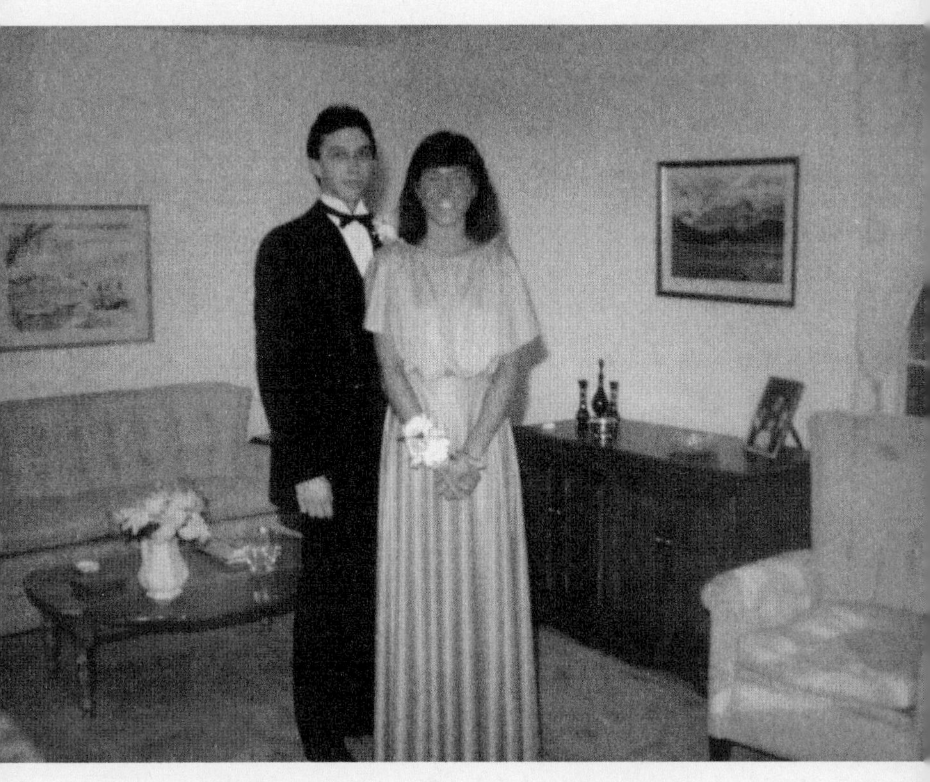

Neal and I headed off to my senior prom, May 1983

24

Break on Through

—The Doors

I was a bit annoyed when the *Washington Post* article came out in May of 2011, but not because I didn't like it. The article itself was terrific! What got to me was the fact that it was written as if *that* was the whole story. To me it was akin to playing one note on a piano and calling it a masterpiece. Jim and I received hundreds of really thoughtful and supportive e-mails from people who had read the *Post* article assuming that this one account included every bit of information that existed about me and my life struggles, as well as those of my family. The events in the *Washington Post* article were just one small part of the story, and because of that, the whole story couldn't really be fully understood or appreciated by people who read it.

Babies are coddled, nursed, and coaxed into childhood. Not me. I was born into a life already in progress. When I came home from the hospital, I was expected to perform my duties as a wife and mother. But how was I really supposed to do that? I was a mother with no memories of her own childhood or her own mother. I could barely read or write, cook or clean. I hadn't the slightest idea how to change a diaper or prepare a bottle. I was a wife with no recollection of love, let alone sex. Without knowing it, I was like an actor playing a role that had been assigned to me. I studied what other wives said and did at parties and mimicked their words and gestures. I cooked and cleaned and shopped, not because I wanted to—not because of any choice I had ever made—but because those things were expected of me. My life became a series of precise rules: make sure you always do this; make sure you never do that.

The old Su may have longed to finish school, to return to work, to seize all the dreams she had left at the door to motherhood. As for me, this was the only life I had ever known. For years, I had nothing to long for. I had no neglected hobbies, no dormant talents, and no dreams that I knew about. I existed for the sole purpose of serving my husband and children. There was nothing else. There was no other me. And, yes, I was content, because I didn't know any better.

For years, I basically just ignored all the things I couldn't do. They simply didn't occur to me, and I didn't have the ability to see myself from anybody else's perspective. People remember their childhoods. I don't. People know how to multiply. Not me. People could talk about what they learned in high school and college. Nope. No high school and no college for me to talk about. People remember their birthdays and how old they are. I didn't remember either, and when I was asked, I would just say the first thing that came into my head. People know how to tie their shoes. There were times when I couldn't. People know how to read and write. Me? Not really. Mothers tell their children what to do and how to act. My children usually told me. Couples love to tell stories of how they met and fell in love, and stories of the crazy things they did in college. I don't have those stories.

It wasn't until we were back from Cairo in the late 1990s that I began to recognize how different I really was from other people, especially other adults. All this time I had thought I was fine. I never saw myself as a freak or as that weird mother. Jim and I never talked about the injury and its consequences because I didn't realize there had been any consequences. Without ever meaning to, I had just been faking it most of the time, especially when I was out around others. For more than twenty years, I have hidden my condition from the world. I had long ago stopped asking everyone to explain the inexplicable. Early on, I had learned to swallow my questions altogether or to only occasionally ask Jim or the kids about stuff I didn't understand. I clung to Jim's side in public, following his cues, speaking only when I was absolutely sure of the right thing to say. Nobody ever seemed to notice or say anything that I knew about or paid attention to. Benjamin, my oldest son (and later Patrick, and then much later Kassidy), became my accomplice in the Meck home, often parenting me and guiding us through the parking lot to our car and through the subdivision to our home, reminding me to take them to school every morning and to pick them up every afternoon. To educate myself, I eventually taught myself to read my children's books and over the years copied a lot of their homework assignments. Benjamin, Patrick, and Kassidy have never once said they thought any of that stuff was weird.

But now I find myself afflicted with a peculiar sort of identity crisis. I don't know who I'm supposed to be. I have spent almost all my life as I know it trying to make other people happy, trying to convince them that I am normal . . . when now I know I am not. I recognize now that I can't act and talk the way other people do. I suddenly feel like such a phony. I was exhausted a lot of the time and terrified of so much because somewhere deep down I was always afraid of being found out.

For twenty-five years, I lived in perpetual fear of sounding stupid, of getting lost, of forgetting what to do or say, of getting caught for being who I really am, of losing my husband and children. I think about things differently now. I get frustrated these days because I don't have any real connection to my parents and siblings. I get irritated with myself for not being able to read and write as I once did. I feel stupid for being unable to sometimes have "adult" conversations, and for getting lost on my way to places I've been to a thousand times. There are so many annoying gaps in my basic comprehension of life that I haven't yet discovered. I still don't even know everything I don't know. And I get incredibly embarrassed. And angry. Angry because I think that no one else can ever really understand what it's like to live this way. Angry because a medical community could see nothing wrong, and thus didn't know how to fix me. And even worse than that, that same medical community assumed there was a psychiatric reason for my condition. No wonder I didn't like talking about it. No wonder I stopped asking questions. I felt like a fraud at times, but it was also clear that nobody was going to tell me how to get back to being the person I once was.

I get asked now if I would ever consider going to see any of these world-famous brain specialists. Pure curiosity would incline me to say, "Yes. Of course." And yet I wouldn't want to be turned into some kind of a human guinea pig. I know now that my condition is considered highly unusual, but maybe it's really not as unusual as people think. Maybe there are many people out there with the same, or at least similar, circumstances as those that I have lived with. Maybe they were told there was nothing that was medically wrong with them, that it was probably all in their heads. Maybe they had doctors tell them that their symptoms were not real. Maybe they have resigned themselves to just getting by as best they can in the world, or worse, maybe they have just given up. Maybe there are people out there who don't have it as good as I had it, surrounded by a supporting family.

Traces of my anterograde amnesia endure to this day. I still experience occasional blackouts, particularly in unfamiliar surroundings, like a hotel room or a friend's guest bedroom. These episodes leave me with entire days of my life that I cannot recall. There are still days when I find myself unable to read or write. And I struggle with the concept of time: I have a hard time putting myself in the future, making decisions about the future, and understanding exactly how far away is next month, or next year. And also the past: how long ago stuff was. I am still forgetful, and I tend to lose memories unless I have a specific reason to retain them, or I write them down. (Jim and our kids used to follow a "three-day" rule: "No matter how badly we screwed up, if we could ride out your wrath or anger or disappointment for three days, you more often than not seemed to forget completely, and it would be as if nothing had ever happened," Jim recalls.)

It is beyond hard to live like I do. Even if I couldn't be "cured" or "fixed," I would be content if some specialist could explain what exactly happened to my brain and why I am the way I am.

Especially if what the experts conceivably found with me could somehow add to the body of brain knowledge and help future head-injury patients and their friends and families to avoid what I have had to go through.

All that being said, a very wise woman, my daughter's professor at Barnard College, Alexandra Horowitz, asked me not long ago, "Su, if there was somehow some magical or medical way, would you really want all your memories back?" My knee-jerk reaction was to say, "Duh! Yes!" But I'm not so sure now. Alexandra said I should instead be happy with the years and all of the memories that I do have instead of languishing over all I don't remember. And that makes a certain amount of sense to me. So many facts, details, people, and places I don't know will, of course, trip me up at weird times, and it really sucks. But if all my memories were somehow restored now, where would that leave me? I would have to figure out exactly who I am all over again. No thanks!

~

And then there is Jim. Jim is obviously not a saint. (Neither am I.) But I have realized it isn't fair to judge him only on the bad stuff he has done. There has been, and continues to be, an awful lot of good stuff, too. Everyone experiences ups and downs in life. Our family's ups and downs have just been a little bit more . . . unusual, and perhaps a bit more extreme. Does *anyone* really know what life has in store? Did Jim know when he married me that he was going to have to at some point show me how to use a toaster safely? Did he realize when he married me he would have to teach me my shapes and colors? Of course not. I can't imagine what it was like for him to wake up with me every morning for *months* after coming home from the hospital and hear me ask him, "Who are *you*?"

Jim is not a bad person. He has done bad things to my kids, and to me, but for me that is somewhat overshadowed by the fact that he has been okay with me telling "the whole story" like this. It speaks *volumes* to me that he would be willing to go on record so that people can begin to understand how devastating a head injury can be to everyone involved. He agreed to put his entire personal life out there right alongside mine because he, just like me, strongly believes it is that important to get the word out about the incredibly destructive nature of brain injuries. Will some people think that I am throwing Jim under a bus? I certainly hope not, because that is not my intention. Why have I stayed with Jim? Dependency? Maybe. He knows me better than I know myself, and even though I know this is going to rub some people the wrong way, I'm just going to come right out and say it: if I didn't have Jim, I wouldn't have me.

That being said, I can't say that I love Jim in the conventional sense that most married couples love each other. I have no idea what it feels like to "fall in love" with another person. I seriously doubt I ever will fall in love, and I am totally okay with that. But the reason for this book was not about a never-ending search for love. I simply wanted to tell my story—the entire story (so far), with all the facts (to the best of my knowledge), in order to, I hope, prevent these things from happening to someone else, or at least to try to help people in similar situations. To be honest, I didn't even know half of my own story when I started this project. Since taking the first steps, I have met and had the opportunity to talk to, so many people who have been instrumental in filling in huge gaps: My immediate family and Neal Moore, of course, but also Kathy, Michele, childhood friends Robin and Diedre, Janet, Valerie, Pam, Jodi, Heather . . .

~

But learning everything about my own life has been secondary to my initial mission. When I began this book project, all I really wanted to do was to explain what it really means to live with a head injury to as many people as would listen. I wanted people to stop saying, "Oh, he just had a concussion. He'll be fine." Or, "Gosh, she's been acting wacky since she bumped her head." I want everyone—parents, spouses, siblings, friends—to start paying attention. I would *love* to get the medical community on board as well. Stop telling people they are crazy. Stop telling people that they can't possibly have forgotten everything just because you—the doctor; the neurologist—don't see anything unusual on an MRI. Please don't tell them that you think they are just seeking attention. Please listen to your patients. Spend more money on brain research. Real research. Discover *new* things. I did.

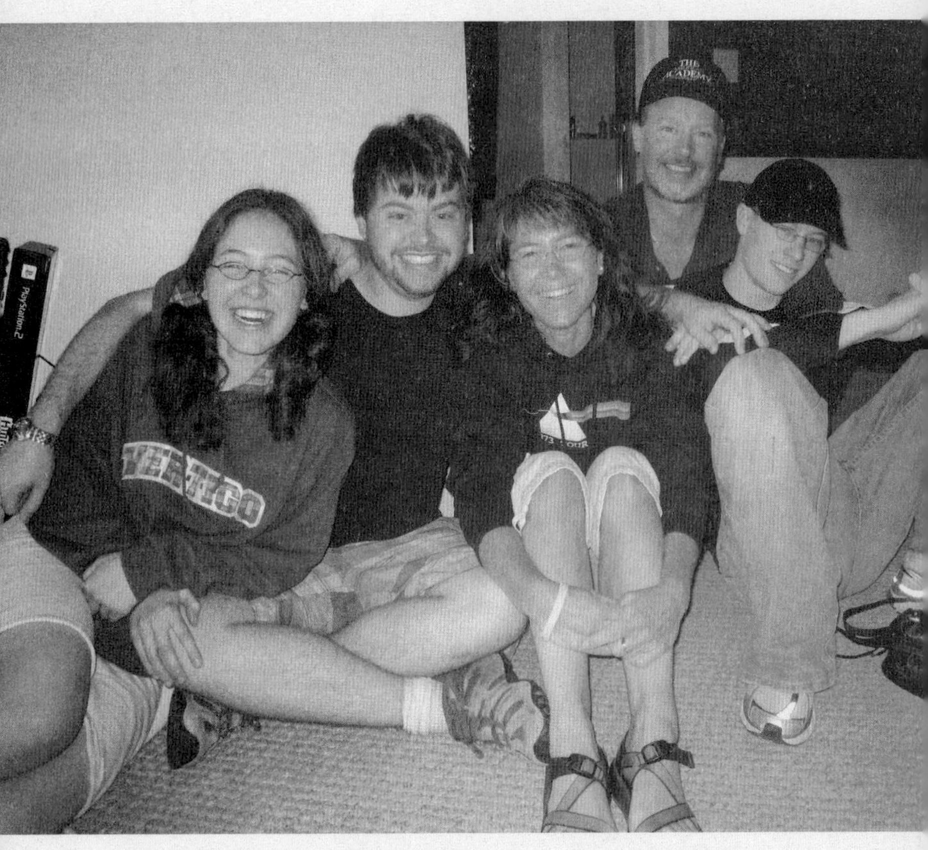

Left to right: Kassidy, Benjamin, me, Jim, and Patrick,
West Hollywood, California, May 2007

Acknowledgments

It's extremely hard to even know where to start! There are so many people who have helped me get to where I am today, but who, unfortunately, didn't make it onto the pages of the final version of this book. The cuts I had to make to this manuscript were positively heartbreaking, but I am hoping that this book is only the beginning. . . . It's true that I don't directly remember anything about, or anyone from, my childhood and teenage years in Mentor, Ohio; Beaver, PA; Wayne, PA; or from my first two years of college at Ohio Wesleyan University. But it is a goal of mine to take a tour someday back to all the neighborhoods where I lived and visit people who may have known me. But until then, I have Facebook, and through it I was able to connect with two of my best girlhood friends and playmates, Robin and Diedre; Lenny, from the Conestoga Marching Band drum line; Laura and Mary, two of my Delta Gamma pledge sisters; and Bob and Paul, two of Jim's fraternity brothers. I have been fortunate that Kathy, one of my best friends from high school, as well as Michele, my sidekick, roommate, and best friend from college, continued to stay in touch with me, even when I had absolutely no idea who they were.

Thanks to Pam Knote, Janet White, Neal Moore, and Valerie Willey for agreeing to be interviewed by Dan. You all helped to shed light on particular details of my story and in turn assisted with the enormous puzzle that is my life.

Special thanks to *anyone* who ever worked with me or took aerobics or Spinning classes from me at any number of clubs where I taught in suburban Maryland both outside Baltimore as well as outside Washington, D.C. I love and miss you all! You all deserve an entire book simply titled *Su: The Strength and Stamina Years.* That being said, I should probably let you all know that, chances are, I wouldn't last through even one class anymore.

To the entire Farrell family, but especially to Imelda. There is a very good chance that I may not have survived without our noontime dog walks together and our enduring friendship.

To countless of my fellow students, faculty, and staff at Montgomery College. You all pointed me in the right direction by giving me the opportunities, encouragement, and confidence that I never knew I had. Again, I thank God (and Mark Zuckerberg) for Facebook and the ability to still keep in touch with so many of you!

And of course to numerous fellow students, faculty, and staff at Smith College. You all know who you are, *and* you should be aware that your book is coming!

Last but certainly not least, to my family. My parents, Bob and Janet Miller; my sister and her husband, Barb and Scott Griffiths, and their daughter, Emily; my other sister and her husband, Diane and Paul Clear, and their kids, Kaitlin, Kevin (and new wife Ashley), and Keenan; my older brother and his wife, Rob and Tracy Miller, and their kids, Amanda, Brandon, and Jake; and my younger brother and his wife, Mark and Tiffany Miller, and their daughters, Morgan and Madeline.

And of course, to Jim and our own kids, Benjamin, Patrick, and Kassidy. This thing was quite an adventure, wasn't it?

Family is always family, no matter what. . . .

I love you all.

~

Dan would like to thank Nick Anderson, his friend and longtime editor, who shepherded the Su Meck story onto the front page; Vernon Loeb, who immediately spotted its book potential; Craig Timberg and Chris Davenport, his *Post* colleagues and friends, who helped explain the whole "book" thing and lent us their agents; Rafael Sagalyn and Gillian MacKenzie, the agents, who provided invaluable advice; Peter Steinberg, who became Su's agent and eventually Dan's as well and represented both of us brilliantly; Jenna Johnson, Valerie Strauss, Bill Turque, Jay Mathews, Michael Alison Chandler, Emma Brown, Donna St. George, and the rest of the current and former *Post* education team, an ensemble with talent to burn; Freddy Kunkle, Craig Singer, John Kelly, Tim Brennan, Chuck Dolan, Skip Sheffield, John Grogan, Neil Santaniello, Bob McCabe, and everyone at GPJams, always ready for another set; Steve Hendrix, Tracy Liden, and Erika Singer, who provided timely guidance in shaping the proposal; Megan Brooks and

Wendell Watson at Texas Health, who helped us find the crucial medical records; Michael Yassa at Johns Hopkins, Daniel Schacter at Harvard, and Larry Squire at UC San Diego, who taught us how memory works; Su's devoted family and friends, who walked us through the missing years; Molly Lindley and Jonathan Karp at Simon & Schuster, who tirelessly, thoughtfully shaped a manuscript into a book; and Su and Jim, the sources who became collaborators and friends. Dan would also like to thank Betty de Visé, his ever-devoted mother; Madeleine and Donovan, his perfect children; and Sophie, his beautiful wife, editor, spiritual advisor and soul mate.

About the Author

Su Meck is pursuing degrees in music and book studies from Smith College. She has high hopes of playing her drums in a local rock and roll band, playing handbells in a New England ensemble, and continuing to sing in community and church choirs. Su wrote a piece for the *New York Times Magazine,* but this is her first book, and she plans to continue writing books while drawing attention to what it is like to live with a traumatic brain injury (TBI). She and her husband, Jim, have three grown children, and currently live in Northampton, Massachusetts, with their two Lab rescue dogs, Fern and Farley, and their two tuxedo cats, Apollo and Athena.

Daniel de Visé is a journalist and author who has worked at the *Washington Post,* the *Miami Herald* and five other newspapers in a twenty-three-year career. He shared a 2001 Pulitzer Prize and has garnered many other national and regional journalism awards; his investigative reporting has twice led to the release of wrongly convicted men from life terms in prison. A graduate of Wesleyan and Northwestern universities, he lives with his wife and children in Maryland. He is working on his second book.

~~J Frankenstein~~